GOOD HABITS FOR HEALTHY KIDS 2-IN-1 COMBO PACK

PROVEN POSITIVE PARENTING TIPS FOR IMPROVING KIDS FITNESS AND CHILDREN'S BEHAVIOUR

BUKKY EKINE-OGUNLANA

CONTENTS

MINI HABITS FOR HAPPY KIDS

Introduction	11
1. Forms of Discipline	17
2. Discipline Without Damage	25
3. Habits to Drill into Kids Early	33
4. Discipline Out of Love	46
5. Creativity Thinking for Kids	60
6. The Right Discipline for Kids	81
7. Problem Handling for Children	94
8. How to Raise Your Type of Child	107
Conclusion	119
References	121

HEALTHY HABITS FOR KIDS

Introduction	127
1. Ways to Encourage Your Child to Be Physically Dynamic	131
2. 7 Styles to Help Get Your Kids to Brush Regularly	137
3. What is Healthy Eating?	142
4. Healthy Drinks for Kids	167
5. Healthy Nutrition For Kids	189
6. Snacks for Kids and WeightLoss	216
7. Healthy Lifestyle For Kids	233
8. Different Games and Activities For Kids	250
9. Heart Healthy Activities For Kids	269

10. Mind-Blowing Exercise Games To Make Kids Active, Fit & Healthy	276
11. Healthy Living Lessons to Teach Your Kids	289
12. Healthy Sleep Habits for Kids	296
Conclusion	309
References	313
Other Books You'll Love!	321

© **Copyright Bukky Ekine-Ogunlana 2020 – All rights reserved.**

The content contained within this book may not be reproduced, duplicated or transmitted without direct written permission from the author or the publisher.

Under no circumstance will any blame or legal responsibility be held against the publisher, or author, for any damages, reparation, or monetary loss due to the information contained within this book. Either directly or indirectly. You are responsible for your own choices, actions and results.

Legal Notice:

This book is copyright protected. This book is only for personal use. You cannot amend, distribute, sell, use, quote or paraphrase any part, or the content within this book, without the consent of the author or publisher.

Disclaimer Notice:

Please note the information contained within this document is for educational and entertainment purpose only. All effort has been executed to present accurate, up to date, and reliable, complete information. No warranties of any kind are declared or implied. Readers acknowledge that the author is not engaging in the rendering of legal, financial, medical or professional advice. The content within this book has been derived from various sources. Please consult a licensed professional before attempting any techniques outlined in this book

By reading this document, the reader agrees that under no circumstances is the author responsible for any losses, direct or indirect, which are incurred as a result of the use of the information contained within this document, including, but not limited to,—errors, omissions, or inaccuracies.

Published by
TCEC Publishing
TCEC House

14-18 Ada Street, London Fields,
E8 4QU, England, Great Britain.

DEDICATION

This book is dedicated to all the wonderful children all over the world who over the years have passed through the T.C.E.C 6-16 year's programme. Thank you for the opportunity to serve you and invest in your colourful and bright future.

MINI HABITS FOR HAPPY KIDS

PROVEN PARENTING TIPS FOR POSITIVE
DISCIPLINE AND IMPROVING KIDS'
BEHAVIOUR

INTRODUCTION

Research shows us that parenting a child with strong self-esteem is more effective than being authoritative. You want your child to listen, admire, and trust you instead of being scared.

All these things are easy to set as targets but challenging to accomplish. *How can you get the balance?*

The dynamics evolve as your child grows, and your views change, but your solution must be constant, intense, and caring. Help your child learn by practice, which helps develop trust and challenges. Calibrate your goals about what your child will do independently, whether you have a child who prefers to sleep through the night, a child who helps put away toys, or an older child who can settle disputes.

As a mom/dad, you can make a strong start of life for your children – they are nurtured, secured, and driven. Parenting is an independence mechanism that teaches your child. As your child grows and evolves, you will do a lot to support him/her. This guide will help you learn more about supportive parenting, stability, and wellness at any point in your child's life.

There is a myriad of techniques that are subject to debate between parents today. Parents find themselves going hoarse as they nag and shout and lecture their children frequently yet see no changes in their behaviour whatsoever. While every child is different, and this book will continue to reiterate that very fact, there are some tried and true strategies that parents can employ in order to improve their disciplining styles.

WHAT DO WE KNOW ABOUT DISCIPLINE?

The term *discipline* comes from a Latin word that means "to teach." As a parent, you are a teacher. How you discipline your kids will help them learn and frame their habits, even as they grow older in age.

For many parents growing up, discipline sometimes meant physical punishment or abuse. It could leave us feeling hurt, angry, and unjustly treated. Discipline is about teaching and guidance. It is a way to keep the kids safe as they grow older and discover more about life. To learn and get on with others, they need to learn how to control their emotions, desires, and actions. Without a doubt, discipline (and teaching the children appropriate ways to act) is one of the most challenging parenting elements.

While there are several different perspectives of how to discipline your child correctly, one concept that is consistent in these many different ideas is that the object of discipline is not merely to make your child behave in the next few minutes or even the same day but to direct your child through their developmental stages while teaching them valuable lessons and behaviours.

Warm but discipline out of love that stimulates the behaviour you want is the best way to train kids. A positive attitude is less challenging for children and makes parenting more fun. It takes time, but, in the long run, it is worth it. It uses love to teach life-long skills rather than fear, and it strengthens the bond with your child.

NURTURING YOUR CHILD

Nurturing is where you need to devote most of your time and effort. Kids learn best once they know they are valued and appreciated. Here are some ideas:

- Love your kids, no matter what they do – and show them you care.
- Listen to your children.
- When they act satisfactorily, praise them.
- Always expect the best of your children.
- Ensure they are safe, both physically and emotionally.
- Finally, be a good role model!

UNDERSTANDING CHILDREN'S BEHAVIOUR

Toddlers sometimes demonstrate their feeling in their behaviour. They are yet to learn the correct responses to say in every situation.

Parents might think the kid is 'naughty' or playing up when they are going through a lot in their mind.

It is essential to understand what influences the behaviour of your child. They will feel less desire to 'act out' or be 'naughty' if you communicate with what is bothering them.

It is easy to assume that you do not have the time to find out what is going on because life is so busy. However, the more time spent figuring out the actual cause of your child's behaviour would mean less time reacting to their misconduct.

LEARNING WHAT IS EXPECTED

Keep in mind that children are not born knowing how to act. They depend on you to teach them in ways that fit their understanding and skill. They need you to calmly and patiently show them what to do. Just as adults learn through practice, you may need to repeat a lesson several times until it becomes a mastery without your assistance.

That is why many parents get disappointed when the child does not get the point or does not break a bad habit immediately. In fact, you should expect this. You should expect that you will be drilling them with the proper behaviour before your child understands it and can master it without the need for your intervention.

After reading this book, please feel free to leave a review based on your findings and how useful the guide was to you. I would be incredibly thankful if you could take 60 seconds to write a brief review on Amazon, even if it's just a few sentences!

1

FORMS OF DISCIPLINE

Disciplining children is a complicated feat that parents are faced with. Deciding on how to effectively manage your child's behaviour that suits both the child and the parents are intense conversations, but incredibly necessary for raising children. It is something parents have to reckon with reasonably early on, as children grow and are met with different social situations and deal with a myriad of new and complicated emotions. For most, acting out is a means of expressing these newly found emotions.

For parents, discipline is one of the many aspects of raising children that often bring about anxiety. Have you ever wondered how you can discipline your kids without being overly cruel or harsh? As it turns out, certain punishments can be a destructive discipline approach for your kids at whatever age they may be.

As parents, we must correct our kid as they grow older in age. Unfortunately, many parents overlook this, perhaps because they are scared to discipline the children. Of course, discipline is not the same as punishment – as many parents have mistaken it to be.

There are plenty of safe and appropriate methods that will educate your children on right from wrong. It is crucial to develop this compass within your children from an early age. It teaches them a myriad of things from responsibility to respect. As a parent, it is your duty to instil these crucial qualities, and while children are young, they will regularly test and push the boundaries.

So that you know, children will point the finger at their parents in the future if they get into trouble for wrong parenting. That is shameful, I would say.

Discipline involves teaching children according to rules to achieve the best behaviour that prepares them for the future. It invokes their brain and helps them function correctly in society. While discipline invokes the thinking mind, punishment impacts the emotional brain. Do you see why punishment could be destructive – especially for kids?

There are several forms of discipline that can effectively aid your children in mitigating their behaviours. Here are a few:

CALL A TIMEOUT

One of the most successful corrective methods available to parents of young children aged two years through elementary school years is timeout. The timeout solution is effective because it prevents the child from gaining attention that could unconsciously perpetuate improper behaviour. Like every other technique – when the kid misbehaves – you must use timeout unemotionally and regularly. Research shows that the timeout works effectively. However, you must understand how timeout works, how timeout is prevented, and what the parent does when the countdown is over.

Timeouts allow children to take a moment to reckon with the feelings that they are experiencing, as well as will enable the parent to take a moment amid the chaos to collect their own thoughts to react calmly and appropriately. Allowing your children a quiet moment to understand why they are being put in a timeout forces them to see why they were wrong and understand that there are consequences to poor behaviour. It's a method that is continuously implemented in households across the globe for its efficacy.

Understanding both your child's role and the role you play is crucial for the success of timeouts. You must prepare to speak to your child and talk them through why they are in this position in the first place. Listen to your children and recognize why they acted in such a way, to begin with. The key to the success of this method is listening and responding.

Some tips for parents on how to maximize timeout include:

- Introduce timeout by 24 months.
- Select the ideal location in the house where there is no access to electronic or digital tools.
- The timeout should last 1 min per year of the child's age to a maximum of 5 min.
- You should completely ignore a child who is in timeout.
- Do not forget to be the timekeeper.
- When the timeout is over, be friendly with them again and start new activities with them.

Similarly, you should avoid hurting your child's self-esteem by infusing shame, guilt, or a sense of loneliness. Ensuring that you are a reliable support system for your child begins here as you show them that despite their mistakes, you will still remain a constant force of guidance. Show them that while making mistakes can sometimes have consequences, the key is not to traumatize them and deny them of parental love.

Although timeout is an effective disciplinary technique, it may not necessarily eradicate the unwanted character. However, it can certainly lessen the frequency by teaching your children why it is wrong, and the consequences they face should they pursue this route. If you do not see any changes, get a consultation, and pray.

THE REASONING OR AWAY-FROM-THE-MOMENT DISCUSSIONS

Discipline requires both teaching good behaviour and modifying unwanted behaviour. In other words, kids need to know both what to do and what not to do. Generally, predicting and avoiding unwanted behaviour is more successful than punishing them for it. An away-from-the-moment conversation will help reduce negative behaviour by giving parents the chance to teach the child the desirable behaviour in advance. This technique is not suitable for use in children below the age of three to four years.

HERE ARE EFFECTIVE DISCIPLINE STRATEGIES:

Model good behaviour. If you want your child to behave appropriately, then let your child see you doing it first. How do you expect your child to behave well if you yourself do not show a model behaviour? You are your child's most excellent role model during these formative years. Reacting appropriately to the various stressors in your life will only reflect in your children.

Use positive discipline. Gone are the days were parents discipline their children with brooms or grounding them in their rooms, nor the threat of getting their gadgets. Today, many now advocate for positive discipline. Reward your child for good behaviour. That will undoubtedly lead to the retention of acceptable behaviour than punishing them for misbehaving.

Listen to them. If you catch your child misbehaving, talk to them, and listen to what they have to say. Find out the reason. Maybe your child is throwing a tantrum because your child is feeling jealous. Talk and listen to them instead of doling out the consequence of the behaviour immediately. Understand that your children are humans too. They experience incredibly complex emotions, especially at such a young age. Talking them through *why* they feel this way is a step in the correct direction to curbing misbehaviour.

Provide consequences. You must clearly explain to your child that there are consequences for every nasty action that they do. For example, you can tell your child that if they do not keep their play area tidy by returning their toys to where they should be after playing, you will store them away for an entire day. This sets them up for life to understand that this is something they will face increasingly as they age.

Be consistent. As a parent, do not waver in your discipline. You need to be consistent in how you deal with your child. You must show your child that you mean business every time they misbehave. If you have enforced a consequence for bad behaviour, make sure that you stick to it and not bail just after a few minutes because you feel pity for your child. Many parents find that this is the most challenging part. But understand that you are disciplining your child for their own good.

Apply redirection. There are cases where a child misbehaves because they are feeling bored. If that is the case for your child, redirect their energy to misbehave into doing something productive. For example, your 4-year old son is messing up his toys, and maybe he needs another thing to occupy him. Try giving him a colouring book and ask him to colour one page. Then check up on him after. Praise him for a good job and tell him to colour another page.

Revaluate age-appropriateness. Some disciplinary actions need to be age-appropriate. For example, you cannot really discipline a 6-year old boy the same way you discipline his 9-year old brother or sister. Keep in mind a child's age when disciplining them as certain punishments will have less efficacy, depending on what age or stage your child is at.

Avoid nagging, yelling, threatening, or punishing. As mentioned, gone are the days of threats and punishments. Countless studies have shown that punishments do not really help enforce good behaviour. It does the opposite instead. The same with nagging, yelling and threatening. These will only push the child to rebel and commit misbehaviour even more.

Many parents have struggled with finding a suitable disciplining style for their children, with many of them trying out different techniques and strategies before finding one that suited their child the best. While consistency is vital, finding an appropriate disciplining method that will have the most profound impact on your child's behaviour is more important. Don't be afraid to try different techniques. Some children respond well to timeouts, while some respond better to having privileges taken away. As your child continues to age, you may need to adapt to how you parent your child as well. The important thing is being receptive to your child's changing behaviours and growth in order to tailor the best methods to them in order for them to learn the correct actions correctly and safely. Know that it may take some time experimenting with different punishments. But once you have found what works best for both you and your child, stay consistent.

2

DISCIPLINE WITHOUT DAMAGE

A child comes into the world with a blank mind: no ideas, philosophy, way to live or act. As they grow up, they depend on the family where they are raised. The parents (or siblings) then teach them and instil doctrines, values, discipline, and more.

Disciplining children is a universal thing that all parents are faced with. Regardless of your religion or culture, parents have the responsibility and duty of instilling the good qualities within their children. This is a universal understanding from the moment a child is born.

I grew up in a Christian home. My parents believed that there is no wisdom in the world except that which is from the scriptures – God's word. According to my parents, even philosophers derive their dexterity and wisdom from the word of God. So, they brought me up with the scriptures' views, and I am such kind of person now. Haha!

The word of God says, "Thy word oh Lord is forever and ever."

The bible is the only book in the world that stays true and shines in all situations. It guides and has answers to whatever life issues and questions anyone might have. And as it is with me, my parents instilled this knowledge in me from my toddler age to always turn to it whenever I need answers to life challenges. Of course, as a man, I cannot look elsewhere. Even now, I meditate regularly, reading and studying the scriptures – that is a habit I learned from my parent!

For me, as a Christian, my parents believed that there is no wisdom anywhere else, but in God's word, all philosophers only derive their philosophy from the word of God. So, the basis on which I was raised was from the book of books, which is from the word of God.

Thy word, oh Lord, is forever and ever. The bible is the only book in the whole world that is true. It has the right answers. If you know where to find it, I was instilled with the knowledge of God's word early so that I should not be looking for answers in a difficult situation later in life because I have been taught where to find answers, developing the habit of reading the bible regularly, meditating and studying the scriptures instils the right pattern into any child and once this has been done early, it is easier to navigate when the child finds him/herself in a difficult situation, the holy spirit will remind the child from what has been put inside.

For example, when Joshua was a kid, his memory was empty: he did not know anything or know life. His parents, however, filled his mind and brought him in the way of the Lord. He also went to the temple to learn from the teachers called "Rabbi." These precepts guided Joshua, and he was diligent in all his deeds, even till age 20. And God walked with him hence.

A child may come from a faulty culture or wrong philosophy. However, instilling the right habits will restore the child and make him readjust to the standard way of thinking or doing things. Discipline sets right and brings a child to his good senses.

Regardless of where a child comes from, understanding that there are societal standards of appropriate behaviour and responses to situations is crucial for their success. A parent's job is to instil these values, regardless of their beliefs. Parents have the freedom to do so; however, they please. Many choose to raise their children as their own parents have raised them. Some, with time and age, have chosen a different path. Despite technology and new parenting methods and trends that have come and gone, what has ultimately remained constant is that we are all human beings who need love as much as we need discipline. Instil this within your children so that they can continue to do the same as they eventually raise the next generation.

Whatever age your child is, between 0-12, keep in mind that you must be consistent in your discipline approach. The reason is if you are not serious, there is a tendency your kids will not take you seriously either.

You could have a blank paper to list ideas as they flow to your mind. After all, your kids will learn what they see you often do. With time, they tend to speak like you, dress like you, and walk like you.

Parents can be a possible climax to which children can arrive. My handwriting, for instance, was from my mum because she taught me how to write. Every child becomes like the parent or teacher who drills habits into them. All your child is emanating from you as a parent is your real you, which is very influential over your children!

INFANTS (BIRTH TO 12 MONTHS)

Infants need to drink, sleep, and play or communicate with others on a schedule. The schedule helps control autonomous functions and gives a sense of security and predictability. It does not overstimulate babies. As a parent, you should allow space for them to grow some resistance to anger and the capacity to self-soothe. You should not use discipline techniques such as timeout, spanking, or consequences.

EARLY TODDLERS (ONE YEAR TO TWO YEARS)

Toddlers are incredibly vocal with their emotions. When they are happy, they demonstrate extreme happiness. The same goes for the opposite emotions. As they are just barely grasping their emotions, toddlers often misbehave as a result of this.

It is common and natural in the early years of a child to play with physical objects and with the ability to exert their own will against others. Parental tolerance is accordingly recommended. To ensure the protection of the toddler, restrict aggression, and avoid disruptive behaviour. Cautioning the child with a "No" face or another very short verbal clarification ("No-hot") and guiding the child to an alternative activity works effectively. During such times, the parent should stay with the child to supervise and ensure that the behaviour does not recur. Moreover, to assure the child that you still love him or her regardless of whatever conduct.

Early toddlers are very vulnerable to feelings of abandonment. You should not keep them away from yourself in timeout. However, sometimes, you can become so upset with the child and may need to set a child's separation period.

Putting it into action: The toddler wants to play with a sharp object, for instance, a knife in the kitchen. Use simple words to try and express to them that they should not be playing with dangerous objects because they can cause harm. Collect the knife and ensure that you have placed it in a safe distance to avoid this from happening again and remove the child away from the environment. As children are incredibly young and small, their concept of time is different, and their attention span can be diverted quickly. Don't harp and linger on the subject for too long. Instead, redirect their attention to a more suitable activity such as playing a puzzle game or ball in another room.

LATE TODDLERS (TWO YEARS TO THREE YEARS)

The search continues for mastery, freedom, and self-assertion. At this age, toddlers are incredibly curious and seek to explore everything within their reach. As they test their newfound independence, your job is to establish the limits. The child's anger at the recognition of limits in such struggles contributes to outbursts of rage. Rage or willful defiance is not usually conveyed in this manner. The caregiver should be empathic, recognizing the importance of these manifestations. As a parent, you should continue to supervise, set boundaries and schedules simultaneously. Set reasonable expectations of the achievement capabilities of the toddler. Knowing how your child reacts helps reduce circumstances in which frustrations flare-up. Also, you should offer a concise verbal clarification and reassurance when the child regains control.

At this stage, children want to explore their independence and tantrums can follow when they are not given what they want in order to nip them at the bud, curb tantrums by leaning into your child's need for a sense of autonomy. Offer them choices, and often two is enough for kids at this age. For example, "What do you want to eat: some fruit or some cereal?"

Minimize meltdowns by being able to anticipate what triggers them. Children are creatures of habit, and you will quickly learn their reasons for having a tantrum often repeats itself. If your child gets upset when they are hungry, prepare ahead of time with several snacks. If they get cranky and overtired, be consistent with a sleep schedule that makes time for plenty of naps.

Your reaction to these meltdowns is just as important as how you deal with them. Keep your cool, no matter how loud or emotional your child gets. Your attention to them is already spurring them on and encouraging them to keep going. Calmly explain to them why behaving in such a way will not give them what they want and is not an appropriate response to any situation.

3

HABITS TO DRILL INTO KIDS EARLY

Most parents know full well that it is much less successful telling children what to do and how to behave than to show them what to do and how to do it. Teaching children a healthy habit early in life works better if parents themselves model their behaviours or behaviour.

Children search for encouragement from their parents, whether they are 3 or 13, so it is fantastic to drill these behaviours in children's early days.

We've all learned how successful people have similar characteristics and how they are the same across cultures and countries. But what if we told you that good parents have the same behaviours, too?

Everyone wants to know the secret of bringing up good kids. After all, no one wants a child that will not give them pride. Right?

There is something to consider before we go any further: **no one is perfect**.

While you strive to be the best parent, you can make mistakes repeatedly. You cannot deny it. This is something that parents face at some point or another. Just as much as they cannot be perfect, neither can their children be. Swallow this pill quickly, because for many parents, it can undoubtedly lead to a fractured and challenging relationship with their children that is fueled by resentment. Fortunately, if you take the right approach, your children will be placed on the road to potential success.

That said, now let us discuss practices to teach your children at the early stage.

CLEAN UP AFTER MEALS

Most children consume their food and sprint from the table afterwards.

They hope that their parents or brother would catch up. You do not want your child to have this bad habit. Instead, show them how to empty their dishes, rinse and place them in a dishwasher (if applicable).

When your child learns this pattern, it is likely to accompany her throughout her entire life, and it is also a transferable skill that will follow them for the rest of their lives, well into adulthood. Instilling a sense of responsibility within your children from these simple tasks will only help them in their future. Additionally, it applies to most good habits they develop throughout their lives.

MAKE THEIR BED

It is easy to wake up in the morning and disregard the bed, beelining for the toilet. Unfortunately, if you let this turn into a pattern, the remainder of your child's life will remain a concern (or maybe until they marry). Help them to straighten their bed, fold up the pyjamas, and set the pillows right. This act will not be perfect on the first day, but perfect is not what we want to achieve now but a habit to be cultivated even if it is not done correctly, but after some time, they will get the right routine.

A teacher once told the story about when Jesus rose from the grave, he folded up his cloth nicely, leaving us all an example to follow John 20:7. This story has helped the children in the class to be tidying their beds without reminders at home.

It will take your child some time to get into this schedule. If you do not let it slip, your kid will go by for a few weeks as part of their day.

Instilling this habit first thing in the morning encourages productivity from the start for your children. It encourages a sense of completing tasks the moment they wake and sets them up for success for the rest of their day as they have breakfast and go to school with a positive mindset. Making your bed might be seen as a frivolous task to many, but it can have incredibly effective psychological effects.

BE ON TIME (NO MATTER WHAT)

It is a concern many adults have, but you want to do whatever you can to secure it early.

You should inform your child how important it is to be on-time (unless it is a real emergency), regardless of what happens. It may not appear to be much stuff at a very early age, but that will change as your child hits school age. Each day, they will have to come to class on time.

This approach is one of the tougher behaviours to teach because some children do not understand time value. Yet, it gets easier for a child to adapt as they mature.

Taking up someone else's time is incredibly rude and tells the other person that you do not value their time. Teaching your children this from a young age sets them up for success as they enter school and eventually, the workforce.

HONESTY IS THE BEST POLICY

Is anything worse than lying? You do not want to have your kid into this poor habit early in life because it will take them into society and the workforce.

You should understand from an early age that integrity is the best strategy for your kids.

Indeed, your child may occasionally be lying, but you can never quit teaching. The more you speak about integrity, the more likely your child will take your advice. All kids come with a clean conscience, and lying will weaken their conscience and emotions if you do not help them.

For many kids, part of testing the boundaries is to lie to their parents and try to get away with it. But as the parent, spotting this may be easier than you might think. Part of raising children is that they grow more creative, and your job is to adapt to this. Your children won't have to lie to you if they can speak to you honestly and truthfully. If you seek to raise honest children, don't lie to them and accept that there will be shocking or scary things that they will share with you. But the worst thing for a parent to do is to judge their children harshly. Your first step is always to take a moment to process the information and then calmly offer advice, a solution, or simply a shoulder to cry on.

SAY "THANK YOU," "PLEASE," "SORRY"

Adults who do not know how to be courteous and respectful of others must have skipped this value at a young age.

Please have your kids in the habit of saying thank you and sorry (including related sentences).

Being gracious and respectful are some of the most basic expectations of a human being. Don't forget to instil these in your children as soon as they can form words. It is an essential requirement of humans to be grateful and apologetic when it is their time to be. Get your children used to thanking others for their time, for favours, or any act of kindness.

Tip: You must take this advice if you want your children to do this. If they see you disrespecting someone, such as your mom, they will start thinking it is all right, and it is not. Reflect the behaviours you expect your children to have.

READING

One of the most effective means of educating and valuing children is to teach. Parents should start reading to their children early every day or before they sleep. A strong reading base allows children to improve their language skills and communication skills in today's culture.

The One World Literacy Foundation says that reading skills are necessary because reading skills strengthen vocabulary, focus, discipline, memory, and develop self-confidence.

Instilling a love for books and learning from a young age will encourage a lifelong journey that is filled with education and creativity from books. When you read to your child, you are encouraging them to think beyond their environment and explore their imagination freely. Furthermore, there are several educational books that you can spend time reading with your children to teach them about more intense subjects that you may be nervous about broaching, such as racism and colourism. While the burden on a parents' shoulders is heavy to educate their children about everything in the world, reaching out to external resources like books are a great way to navigate through these topics.

> "A person who does not read has no advantage over a person who cannot read."
>
> — MARK TWAIN

STAYING ACTIVE

Another necessary behaviour is to be involved. Go out and play games and sports with your child. Cycle together and show them the value of fitness and being involved in a healthier life. Active children are less likely to have obesity or sleep disorders.

Furthermore, stop being a couch potato. Offer the kids a chance to participate and train school teams for a safe life.

Our health is something we take for granted, often before its too late. Teaching your children the importance of taking care of ourselves, while instilling a sense of self-love is incredibly complex and a huge responsibility that parents have to bear, but it is necessary. Many eating disorders stem from childhood habits that compound and develop in full force by adulthood. Curbing this by enforcing acceptable practices and a positive way of perceiving their own body is a strategy in combating this.

Remaining Positive

Children will quickly get down if things do not go as they want. To learn to be flexible when faced with losses or sacrificing something is a beneficial skill or pattern in early learning. The "strength of positive thought" creates self-esteem and contributes to a happier and productive future.

RESPECT

Children should learn to treat others early, including their elders, friends, and even animals. You see how your parents handle servers in restaurants or men who sort the garbage, and you benefit from these experiences. Being kind and respectful to others is a tradition that serves you when you get older.

Some people are bullying and shaming in today's online world, and children who have been polite from a young age will help break the loop.

Respect goes beyond merely treating your neighbours with kindness. Respecting oneself is just as important. Teaching your children to be kind to themselves in a world that will continuously have several hostile forces attacking them is crucial for raising confident and strong children. Allowing them to treat themselves with kindness and love is critical to them projecting the same attitude onto the people around them.

HONESTY

Say the facts once. Using errors and acknowledge the consequences. Integrity and dignity will continue with children all their life if their practices are practised early enough.

While understanding the nuances of lying, that will not harm others is something that your children will have to grapple with as they age, understanding that "honesty is the best policy" is the first step to raising healthy children—ensuring that your child has a good relationship with you is how to impart a trusting and honest relationship between parent and child. This way, you will always be aware of what your child is experiencing (particularly mentally) and be able to respond accordingly.

> "Always do good. It will impress others and amaze others."
>
> — MARK TWAIN

GRATEFULNESS

Children will often compare what their peers have and do not. Teach kids to be grateful for what they have in life and make them realize that there are still people who are less than they have. Learning early in life to count your blessings is a journey towards a quiet and peaceful life. It is a lesson that adults still face today, yet instilling this early on teaches your children to quickly face it and internalize the fact that this is the reality that they are faced with, where many people are better off than others, some seemingly so. This is where you attempt to educate your children on complicated topics like materialism and money in a simplified way. It can be extremely daunting, but even so much as trying already places you in the right direction.

FAMILY TOGETHERNESS

Provide as many reminders of the importance of the family as possible. Dinner together, exchange holidays with family members and allow them to be close to their relatives and friends wherever possible.

For many, we take our family for granted. We often assume that they will always be there, but this fantasy comes crashing down as we grapple with changing tides and the journey of life. Teaching your children to value family will only help them appreciate what they have at the moment. The concept of this is difficult for most kids to understand, especially depending on the age group. But spending time with your family and allowing them to experience your family members to the fullest and create beautiful memories is the best way for you to supply your children with a positive outlook on their family.

CLEANLINESS

A simple practice of brushing your teeth twice a day and learning how to flip holds your child's oral health in check. Brushing the teeth at night helps prevent bacteria from feasting on left pieces of food throughout the night. Flossing is incredibly important to manage plaque buildup and take care of your oral health. Showering or bathing and careful handwashing are healthy practices every day to establish early in life, for children. Hygiene is not always understood to be a top priority. When left to their own devices, children will get messy and dirty quickly. Teach your children to consistently practice healthy habits of hygiene in order to present themselves. Not only does this benefit them and the people around them, but it also helps their overall health.

FINAL THOUGHTS

This chapter is just a handful of the many routines that your young children can learn. When you have a plan in action, you need to commit to it if that is what it takes. Within a few days or weeks, some children develop healthy behaviours, while others battle for months. However, if you continue, things will quickly come together.

A last piece of advice. Travel with your children as much as possible to think about new cultures as well. Travelling exposes your children to the scope of how big the world is and offers them new perspectives and outlooks on life and the world. It encourages them to learn more about different environments that create more tolerant and empathetic children.

When you fly, the children get to see a more expansive world view, making them happier citizens. It gives them a greater sense of how much the universe has to offer.

4

DISCIPLINE OUT OF LOVE

How can you teach your child consistency so that they can perform better at home and in public? Parents need their children to be safe, compassionate, respected, and willing to find their place worldwide and as well-behaved adults. Nobody needs to be credited with parenting a spoiled brat.

But often, these expectations seem to be miles away from the actual actions of your infant. Talk on obstacles to good behaviour, successful strategies of supervision, and aid in unsafe activity habits.

One thing that parents tend to forget is that they were children once too. Recall your own childhood and where you feel your own parents lacked or succeeded in when it came to raising you. Be reflective of yourself as you are your child's most outstanding role model.

ESTABLISH YOUR ROLE AS A PARENT

As a parent, you must help your child become self-sufficient, compassionate, and self-controlled. Families, teachers, churches, clinicians, health providers, and others can be beneficial. But parents remain the main burden for control.

The American Mental Health Association defines three parenting models – authoritarian, permissive, and authoritative. What is yours?

An authoritarian parent has reasonable goals and implications for his or her kids.

The influential parent requires versatility and mutual treatment of behavioural problems with the infant. Studies show that this is the most effective method of reproduction.

An oppressive parent has strong goals and ramifications but displays little love for his child. The parent might say things such as, "It is why I am the mum." This is a less successful type of parental education.

On the other hand, a permissive parent displays great love for his or her child but gives no discipline. This is a less successful type of parenthood.

Your children have to understand that while you are a trusty support system that will always be a constant force in their lives, they also have to be able to establish boundaries between parent and child. Finding that balance is often a challenge for many parents because as much as you want to be your child's best friend, you also cannot be a "yes man" which hinders their growth as a person.

DISCIPLINE TECHNIQUES

You can relate the type of unpleasant behaviour your child exhibits by their age, temperament, and, sometimes, your parenting style.

The American Academy of Pediatrics and the American Association of Child and Adolescent Psychiatry prescribe the following:

Good behaviour reward: The only way to inspire the child to proceed is to appreciate good behaviour. In other words, "Catch him as well." Compliment until your kid demonstrates the action that you were hoping they would do.

Social consequences: The child does something wrong, and you caused the child to feel the result. You do not have to "read." The kid cannot blame you for what happened. For example, if a child intentionally damages a toy, they do not get the toy.

Logical consequences: This approach is analogous to natural effects but explains the children's inappropriate actions. The effect is strongly connected to the behaviour. You warn your boy, for example, that if he does not clean up his toys, the toys will be confiscated for a week.

Removing privileges: There is often no rational or natural implications for incorrect actions — or you have little time to worry about it. In this case, a right can be revoked as a result of unacceptable actions. For example, if a middle schoolgirl does not finish her homework on time, her privileges can be taken away during the night. This technique of restraint works well if:

- In any manner, it connects to their actions
- The kid needs everything
- Taken as soon as possible after improper conduct (especially for young children)

Timeouts: Time outs work if you know what the kid did wrong or if the child's behaviour must be changed. Make sure you have a timeout place in advance. It needs to be calm, boring place-perhaps, not a bedroom or a risky area such as a bathroom (where the child will play). This discipline method will work on children while the infant is young enough to appreciate the intent of spending time- usually around two years and older. Time-outs also work well for younger children who view separation from their parents as a loss.

Why spanking and other forms of physical discipline do not work. Here is why:

- Spanking teaches kids that it is okay to hit when they are angry. You want to strive to teach your children anger management techniques, rather than more ways to lash out and negatively handle emotions.
- Spanking can physically abuse your kids or hurt them, which ends up having the effect of instilling fear in them, rather than building trust between the two of you.
- Instead of loving you or changing their misconduct, spanking makes them fearful and teaches them to avoid getting caught of their misdeeds. It fosters secrecy and ways to get around you.

TIPS FOR MAINTAINING DISCIPLINE

In all you do, ensure to direct your teaching to match the temperament of your kid. The secret to successful discipline is to consider your child, particularly his or her temperamental style, and use your discipline to help them reach their potential. However, it should not be your intention to let them him into doing something against their own will.

Say the punishment strategy. Discipline strategies are not meant to come "out of the blue," mainly when you try something new. When dealing with old enough children to grasp, explain the method during a scheduled conversation (not in the heat of the moment), why you are doing what you are doing, and what you intend it to achieve. Older children should be included in the option between incentives and consequences. Never act out of anger. Taking a breather to collect your thoughts and let your children simmer with what they have done is a positive thing for both parent and child.

Love your kids. Be compassionate. When you demonstrate respect for your child – significantly though your child is punished – your child will be more likely to respect you, your family members, and those in your own life. Apologize when you "lose it" or overreact in contempt. Act like them sometimes, if that works.

Be clear. Any strategy can fail if you do not systematically obey or apply implications. For example, if you claim your toys are out of limits for a week, take them away if the offending activity persists.

Avoid the lecture. While you may be incredibly disappointed by your child, save the long-winded lecture. Especially when they are younger, simply putting why you are disappointed by their actions and what they should do next time instead would suffice. Long-winded speeches often confuse children. You want to be clear and concise.

Do not crack the control. Do not give in by offering negative conduct in public events, such as a kid who throws a tangle while shopping. If you disagree with the demands of the kid, the tantrums will proceed. Know that the behaviour will pass and your child will be back to their happy selves, provided that you supply them with the right discipline.

Work to keep the priorities and methods intact over time. If more than one parent is responsible for the infant's discipline, please make sure that you compromise on the techniques.

It has not been done until it is done. Help your child come back to a suitable game.

Understand what is best for the growth of your child. Ensure that the kid fully knows what you wanted him or her to do before disciplining the infant. Parents often expect action which goes beyond the capacity of the child to obey. As with all essential life tips, behaviour also needs time for a frame-up.

Look for the "why" behind actions. When you see an unacceptable behaviour trend, part of the remedy is to search for "whys." For example, your child may be frustrated about something else or a friend leaving. Perhaps your child had a rough school day. Maybe your child is overwhelmed by family issues.

This does not explain the behaviour, but it allows you and your child to find ways to avoid it from repeatedly happening by seeking to explain why it happens.

Give time to relax and cool down. Sometimes, your child may do something that just really ticks you off. Instead of immediately reacting and scolding your child, give yourself a moment to cool down. Lie down and relax first. If you respond immediately to your anger, there is a greater chance that your anger will cloud your judgment.

Settle everything before bed. Try to settle matters before you go to bed. This will make sure that problems are dealt with as soon as possible. Just like we said earlier that brushing the teeth helps stop bacterial from feasting on little pieces of leftover food, in that same way, sorting things out before you sleep helps prevent anger from festering on the mind through the night. Going to sleep with everything resolved allows for the next day to be a fresh start of good behaviour. However, this does not apply to all problems because some need both parties to cool down and are best dealt with the morning after. Some issues are more complicated than others. But always bear in mind to try to resolve things before heading to sleep.

Create meaningful "heart-to-heart" moments. When you see your child often misbehaving, seat the child down, and talk to them about it. It is always better to settle issues with a good heart-to-heart talk, especially on sensitive issues. If you think that your child needs coaxing to let what they are feeling out, then you must initiate the conversation yourself. Be open and vulnerable to your child. This does not mean lay all of your own adult problems onto your children, but relate to them and express to them that perhaps you might have been frustrated today as well, but instead of taking out your anger by screaming and having a tantrum, you chose to deal with it calmly and rationally. Your children lead by example and having an adult that they can model their behaviour after. As your children age, perhaps the conversations can grow more serious and reflect the realities of the world. But in the meantime, while they are extremely young, don't be afraid to open up a little bit as well.

Use examples. When you try to discipline your child and teach them a lesson on something, try to use examples that they can relate to themselves. For example, if you want to teach your child the discipline of brushing their teeth every night, you can say, "if you don't brush your teeth before bed, you are allowing the germs to feast on your mouth, and you will lose your teeth." Sometimes a good bedtime story with discipline is a good trick.

KNOW WHEN AND WHERE TO GO FOR HELP

Give yourself a rest once you have the best discipline and style. There are days when nothing seems to fit. Maybe you had a bad day, too. It needs a lot of preparation and effort to develop skills for construction management. Be frank with yourself if you believe like you have made an error. Excuse your child and explain to the child how the next time you will expect to alter your answer.

Often you do not know what to do next. Parents are faced with a number of choices and the constant pressure of messing up that they panic and have moments of anxiety. Or you do not know how to alter anything more successful than what you are doing now. Perhaps you feel like you have hit a roadblock in your child's development and want more advice on how to proceed.

Whenever you have concerns about your child's actions and instruction, pray to God, and consult with your child's doctor. It could be time for a health specialist to support you whenever you see:

- A lack of regard or respect for other authorities such as guardians, teachers, and other adults in general.
- Actions that have been taught to be offensive or damaging, yet your children persist with this behaviour.
- Signs of despair, extreme sadness, lack of motivation long-term blueness, loneliness or lack of motivation. Sometimes the symptoms are not so clear and forward.
- Your child uses medications, drugs, or alcohol to treat depression or other life issues.
- Several family ties are complicated. Volatile relationships can affect your children negatively that they act out as a result in order to deal with the intense emotions they are experiencing.

FIVE GOLDEN RULES OF DISCIPLINE

Stand firm. We all hate confrontation, but if you do not obey the rules and repercussions you have created, your kids will not do so. It is that simple. So, do not waver in your decisions. If your kids see that you cannot hold on to the rules that you set yourself, they will not put importance on that rule and will eventually "slip up" and do it again. Or they may see it as a sign that you are not a strong authority figure in their life which allows them to act out and not afford you with the respect you deserve.

Pick your battles. Give little things little attention and big stuff much focus, and you are happy and calmer — and (bonus!) the kids are healthier, more relaxed, and stronger, too. You must remember that not every misbehaviour warrants your focus and vigilance. If you take notice of every little mistake that your child commits, you will end smothering your child. When children get too "smothered" with how you are, they tend to misbehave even more. So, give your child a break and focus only on their misbehaviours and mistakes when it is truly despicable. Remember that children are constantly testing the boundaries. For you to react strongly to every act of mischief and dole out punishment can take a toll on your own mental health as well.

Praise, do not punish. Continue to exercise mindfulness of positive feelings. Do not administer any punishment as that has already been proven to be a moot point. Instead, practice praising and positive feedback. In other words, your tone of voice, your actions, your vocabulary ought to sound good 80% of the time with your child. This act even works well as you cannot get it wrong. But although your voice is pleasant, do not forget to stay firm still. Most children want to be praised and be told that they are good and have made the right choices. Implement this in your parenting style because positive reinforcement is a force that really plays a profound impact on your child.

Set clear rules and expectations. A thoroughly chosen set of age-appropriate rules will make family life even simpler and cleaner, says Radcliffe. For instance, the "no cookies before dinner" rule avoids daily snacking claims before dinner. The "no machine after 10 p.m." law avoids a nighttime contention about the shutdown of the pc. You need to set up clear expectations of the rules with your kids. Do not provide room for misinterpretation as sometimes kids can exploit that to get their way. Maintain simplicity when setting the guidelines for your children. While expectations can be complex, it doesn't have to be for your kids.

Provide unconditional love. Yeah, it is a no-brainer, but kids need to know that every day, even though they have done something wrong, you love them. Show your kids that you love them despite the fact they misbehave systems. This will help your kids understand that you are fair to them and that what you are doing is for their own good. Despite the disciplinary consequences in place, make sure your children know that it comes from a place of love and care for them. Always make sure to spend time with your kids after the punishment to convey that all is forgiven. As you help your child grow and go through their own journey of life, you are a support system that will always provide them with the love they deserve.

CREATIVITY THINKING FOR KIDS

Were you aware that you are creative? Even if you do not think your child is talented, God has made everyone exceptional and beautiful. God is the creator of all humans, and we are all made in his image and likeness. He encourages us all to use our imagination to make the world a better place. Moreover, we are a representation of him.

As humans, we often think of imagination as an innate trait or, sometimes, a learned skill. That is a very wrong concept: no one was ever-talented by birth. However, parents should encourage the imaginative thinking skills of their children at an early age. This can be instilled through a myriad of ways that may not be the most conventional either. Creativity stems from several methods and simply getting your child's brain thinking is already an act of exercising their creative skills.

Although you cannot promise that your child will become the next Picasso, you can give them a leg, giving them all the support, they need for imaginative thought. Activities such as arts, building blocks, and creative play will help the children develop their understanding and creativity.

Here are also various suggestions which will help parents encourage imaginative thinking and spending time with children.

EXPLORE SPACE

Learning about outdoor space often catches children's interest, so it can be a perfect way to inspire their creativity while allowing them the opportunity to venture into science lessons.

Furthermore, you can do many educational and imaginative things to stimulate your boy's fun activities for space.

Some of these exercises are very simple. You may encourage your child to use their imagination to tell you, for instance, what they believe the aliens are or ask them to tell a story about an astronaut who flew to the Moon.

You should also do creative exercises more deeply to inspire your child to learn about space. Solar panel paper mâché models are a perfect art activity for children, and Styrofoam balls will also render models.

Planetariums are another perfect way for your children to interact in nature. Planetariums also host fun movies and children's events to learn more about outdoor space. These outdoor excursions are an exciting way to spend time with your children. Science centers are another great way to learn about space, among a slew of other subjects like animals and chemistry. These centers are explicitly made to enrich your child's learning experience and go above and beyond to provide activities and learning opportunities with the number of experts and educators that are available at these centers.

These excursions apply for all ages, and parents often find themselves enjoying their time and learning a thing or two as well. While outings like these are not a common thing, they are a great way to treat your children and reward their good behaviour. They are also a great way to get out of the house and cater an outing specifically to your child that they will enjoy.

There are also plenty of online resources that are reliable and trustworthy for educating your children in a fun way.

For example, the NASA website is widely used by kids as it has an entire subsection dedicated to educating children with fun games, interactive videos and activities. Instead of spending their afternoons watching TV, perhaps take some time to sit together and explore these resources. There are several teacher-approved apps and websites that are recommended to enhance a child's learning further.

Encouraging your child's passion for open space through art and their creativity will help you build your home for your child. Space captures children and inspires them to try and visualize the wonder that exists outside of Earth, which is why it is so popular among children. The stars, planets and possibility of aliens capture children and exercises their brains to think outside of the box and outside the realm of possibilities. Studying space is a fantastic way to foster logic while also encouraging creativity in your children.

MAKE GIFTS

How do you let your children pick presents for their families as the holidays roll around?

Can you pick something tiny in the shop, or do you only have them in a package you have chosen?

If you want to do something else this year, your kids should make donations for others rather than buy something from the shop. Whereas the presents from shops bought by adults and youth are often well-thought-out, children's gifts often feel like an afterthought, unless handmade.

Creating presents for your children to send them to family members may be an ideal way for you to teach your children the value of offering presents. Unlike a small drink or card signature, it is a more intimate opportunity for the children to appreciate their friends and relatives.

Small beverages – such as bracelets or ornaments – are lovely and ideal creations for children of all ages, and you have much space in which to develop designs. You can paint wood ornamentations, learn how to braid friendship bracelets, or make adorable and unforgettable presents for your children by creating your snow globe kits.

When children grow older, they could choose to create advanced and customized products for the people they love. They can paint portraits of areas that your family loves, or they can carve, model, or craft more technical woodwork.

Gifts are a perfect way to foster ingenuity while allowing children to grow socially. Gift-giving is a great way to teach, especially younger children kindness and how to share their things. As your children age, they will love creating things that they are proud of that have a purpose for someone else.

They will want to share their talents and share the joy with those around them, which is why gift-giving is often met with such enthusiasm from children.

It is also a great way to spend time with your children. Arts and crafts are a fantastic way to get your child using their hands and tools while tapping into their tactile side to make a product that they have envisioned, planned for and executed.

MAKE TOY CRAFT KITS WITH YOUR KIDS

Toy craft kits are another perfect way to encourage creative ingenuity.

The kits are great opportunities to help your child practice their imagination while developing their fine motor skills. As an extra benefit, they can learn how to make things using their two hands.

Toy craft kits are available in all types. For younger children, you can do basic, easy-to-make, and personalize toys like pinwheels and tops. Easy and exciting science and craft kits are also available.

More complicated tasks might be appreciated for older children. You may want to make your own tea set or pound set, or you may want to make a model ship or train. You may get exciting chemistry kits or necessary devices for technologically inclined children.

Since there are so many toy craft kits online, you can easily find one that attracts your child, perfect for their ability level. There are also plenty of inexpensive options that can be found at variety shops. If these are also unavailable to you, purchasing inexpensive materials to come up with your own kit might take a little bit more effort, but will induce hours of entertainment and creativity for your child.

For more fun, make a family art project in which all your family members pitch. A birdhouse, a children's table, or other larger craft is one of the best ways to shape a family bond. These are great ways to get your children involved with nature and their outside environment as well. Remember that almost anything can be made into a child's playground. It's genuinely about how enforcing a positive attitude even towards the littlest things and encouraging your children to explore.

ENCOURAGE KIDS TO USE BUILDING TOYS

Design toys, such as blocks and Legos, can be fantastic opportunities for children to explore and expand their creativity.

You should give plenty of time for free playing with construction toys with your kids, but you should also challenge them to build something of interest to them. For example, if your 8-year-old likes cars, you could have a Lego car set and allow them to make a dream car.

You would have to consider a strategy that works to achieve what you want and set a realistic target. This principle helps your child practise their problem-solving skill while improvising to build the product of their dreams.

During free play with toys, your children can extend their imagination and play with objects. A little child might enjoy building a city with blocks to play with toys, and older children will enjoy building sets based on their favourite television and movie characters.

You should give your children plenty of space for fun, creative play with building toys, but you should also challenge them to keep them interested and aware. These obstacles should usually be opened to ensure that children continue to use their imagination. This style of toy is an ideal way to help your child grow their motor skills and spatial skills. They stimulate the imagination as they build simple to intricate shapes and also when they are demolishing their builds. Building toys encourage your children to think logically while also having a vision in mind that they are seeking to execute. This is a great skill that will accompany them as they age and enter school, and eventually, the workforce where problem-solving is crucial for every adult's life.

USE APPS, GAMES, AND GADGETS

Parents often ask the question, "Does technology limit innovation?" The answer is NO. Technology does not limit or affect a child's innovation in any way. Although spending too much time in front of the TV or some set of toys may be wrong.

However, using technology appropriately and in balance will improve children's innovative reasoning skills through software, games, and gadgets.

Many brain-boosting memories games and software out there are designed to help improve kids' memory in a fun and entertaining way. They help exercise your child's brain, improve concentration, enhance cognitive function, boost focus and attention.

Brain games will stimulate your child's thinking ability in unconventional ways to solve a problem. The benefits of brain games are numerous as they improve your child's memory and decision-making skills, as well as reaction control and their focus. Like physical exercise, the brain needs stimulation to improve upon analytical thinking, creativity, and problem-solving. The best part is that kids are likely to be open to the idea of a game as compared to, say, reading books. A brain workout for kids encourages a number of practical skills like planning, visual attention and employing some logic or math skills.

Similarly, language applications can help kids learn a second language. Learning a second language, especially at a young age, is extremely beneficial as children at this age are like sponges where they soak up new information far more quickly than an adult would. Encouraging a second language opens up a myriad of benefits as it exposes them to a new culture, new experiences and can significantly benefit them in the future. Learning languages also do not have to be intense practice unless they wish it. It can be as simple and as casual as simply watching cartoons in a different language or playing games in their target language.

Contrary to the assumptions of many parents, video games are not negative news for your child. If you choose to engage in age-appropriate games, they will improve your child's ability to believe and solve challenges creatively. You should also encourage your kids to play with various devices to relax and be curious about technology. This is also an excellent opportunity to educate your children on proper internet etiquette. Teach them about the dangers that lie outside of their bubble while also ensuring that parental locks are in place to manage their internet usage responsibly.

Gaming equipment, telescopes, and toy robots are beautiful tools that allow your children to explore technology to their imaginative thinking. Therefore, technology can be a fantastic way for children to stretch their imaginative powers, but parents can still be aware of how long their children are on the computer.

Although art apps or video games can help enhance fine motor skills and increase children's capacity to overcome challenges, they cannot replace real-life activities. While parents cannot focus on technology, it can be an excellent tool to build an exciting and creative atmosphere at home.

COOK WITH YOUR KIDS

It is undoubtedly overwhelming for children to cook. It is an opportunity to teach them a great life skill by improving their ability to solve problems creatively.

If your children are young, begin with essential recipes such as baked goods. It is easy to make muffins, cookies and loaf cakes like banana bread. For recipes of this nature, there aren't too many steps your young ones will need to adhere to. Plus, if you run out of milk or eggs, you will expose them to the idea of substitution and different techniques and methods for problem-solving in the kitchen. Exposing them to the kitchen from a young age ensures that they are not intimidated by the kitchen as they age and will be motivated to try cooking when they reach older ages.

As your children grow older, you could expose them to complicated recipes that require more abilities to prepare. For instance, you can begin with Cottage Pie then to a more complex Boeuf Bourguignon recipe. Encourage them to try new foods and find recipes that excite them. Allow them to take the reins and offer minimal help unless asked. Give your children the chance to spread their wings and flourish in new territory. While mistakes can happen, guide them to make sure they are practising safe habits.

Although it will take longer for your children to eat in the kitchen, watching them learn and grow up would be worthwhile. Besides, cooking is an experience that you will enjoy with them even though they might be adults at that stage.

Getting your children in the kitchen is a great way to encourage independence and teach them skills that are important for the future. If your children are picky eaters, in particular, getting them involved with cooking and baking can show them to be unafraid of new foods and flavours. It can get them excited to eat as they have a hand in the process of creating the final product. You will not only offer your children an invaluable skill to use later in life, but it will also help develop their capacity to think creatively, solve challenges, and handle resources.

MAKE ART WITH YOUR KIDS

Making art for your children is one of the easiest ways of turning your home into a fun, artistic space.

Kunst is an effective way for children to express themselves and develop their artistic skills. It improves your motor skills and encourages you to expand your creativity.

You should still ensure that you have art supplies in your house. You do not have to buy a Hobby Lobby, but some pencils, Play-Doh, and coloured paper will help inspire your children to make use of their imagination regularly. These tools are inexpensive but can inspire your children to create pictures and projects that allow them to express their creative side. Fostering this habit will enable them to think outside of the box and come up with their own original ideas.

You can also create art projects for your baby. While you may not be an artist, you should indeed teach your child basic crafts such as making flowers from tissues and pipes or making festive paper chains.

Signing up your children for art lessons with your child is another beautiful way to communicate with your child while art is being made. Parent-kid pottery lessons are a disorderly yet enjoyable way to communicate and build with your kids, and you should use these classes as a chance to practice together if you are not the most skilled artist.

You will let them develop their imagination by making art with your children while improving their ability to articulate themselves and travel carefully.

TEACH THEM HOW TO PLAY MUSIC

Another perfect way to inspire innovation at home is to play music with your children. Music is a well-loved extracurricular that parents all around the world encourage their children to pursue. It fosters a discipline and a sense of responsibility. It also increases memory skills and improves their coordination. Having an education in music teaches your children to persevere and as they meet the goals that they have set for themselves, gives them a sense of achievement. It is also another effective way to nurture self-expression.

If your child is an only child, you can assist with this by giving them necessary instruments like kids' keyboards and drums, and you can even enrol them in music lessons targeted at children.

As your children step closer to adulthood, you should teach them the fundamentals or enrol them in beginner lessons for simple instruments like the piano.

Children from primary school will have plenty of chances to participate in music when they grow older. Schools will also have music lessons for children singing and playing a recorder, and your children should enter music clubs.

Your kids will also be part of the school band, chorus, or orchestra if they want to play different instruments and practice music.

Even when your kid is not close to nearby Mozart, you must teach them how to play music to learn about their talent and cultivate their love for good music.

MAKE A PHOTO BOOTH

Taking a photo booth is a perfect way to dress up, offer photography to girls, and at the same time, make invaluable memories.

You can begin by collecting old clothing, fun costumes, and fascinating tips around your home by making a photo booth for your children. While you should still purchase things that your children like, you should be sure to find many dress-ups at home.

You can visit the nearest thrift store if you need a few additional supplies. Thrift shops are often packed with fun-and cheap-items to wear while your children are dressed.

Next, you can build a picture area for your children. You can clear a specific wall or hang a sheet for a lovely backdrop, and you can catch some lamps to boost lighting in any room.

Then dress up and snap away from your children! If your children are old enough, you can show them how to use the camera, and you can also involve them in the setup.

You will have a set of pictures at the end of the picture, put in your scrapbooks, and save them for when they are older, and your kids will have fun.

Creating a photo booth is the best place for your children to make lasting memories and be imaginative.

Some children might prefer to be on the other side of the camera, so always consider the flipside as well. In this case, teaching your children the essential functions of a camera and then allowing them to use their creativity and imagination to take pictures as they see fit is a great way to foster another hobby from a young age.

GO ON CREATIVE "MINI FIELD TRIPS"

Small businesses in areas that foster innovation will help connect your child to fresh and exciting experiences. Encourage outings with your children to explore your local areas. Go on walks and explore the nature that surrounds you. This way, your child becomes more acclimated with spending time outside, gets plenty of fresh air and exercise, and is more in tune with nature, which has its own way of relaxing a person.

Museums are a convenient and cheap way to inspire innovative thought. Children's museums also have a wide range of displays suitable for children and are packed with enjoyable, hands-on experiences that allow your child to experience the world around them.

Other museums, such as art museums or museums of natural history, are also excellent opportunities for youngsters. Although your children should be old enough to grasp the museum's etiquette, these types of museums are perfect examples of teaching your child and stimulating your mind.

Theatre shows are just another fun experience when encouraging your children's artistic climate. Age-appropriate plays and musicals are great opportunities to get the children into theatre, and many children's theatres offer children's acting lessons.

The library is another excellent place for children as there are often sections dedicated for children that feature books, computers and reading corners explicitly designed for entertaining and educating your children. For a bit of quiet time, consider going to the library where your children can pick up their favourite book. If your child has a little bit more energy and is unable to focus, read-alongs are often planned events at libraries that are free to join and a fun way to spend your child's afternoon.

You may also participate in concerts and symphonies to improve your child's music's passion and enjoyment. If it is classical music or a successful singer, your child will grow their talent at live music events. This is a great way also to show your children how music can be transformed in a concert environment. Many musicians and artists have been created in these spaces, where at a young age, they witnessed performances and felt inspired to pursue the arts in the same way.

You can also check at local activities and see if your children can be involved in nearby exhibitions or as speakers. Excellent theatre and history can be enjoyed for your kids at events such as Shakespeare in the park and Renaissance events. Exhibitions on Ancient Egypt or space shuttles can be fantastic opportunities for them.

It becomes apparent that there are hundreds of ways to improve children's imagination, and most of them do not take time. When considering an after-school service, parents should not even have to assist in the curriculum process. Therefore, never fail to inspire children to improve their creative ability, as innovation in the modern world is key.

ORGANIZE STUFF AT HOME WITH YOUR KIDS

You do not have to go far to build a relationship with your kids and enhance their creativity as well. You can do that just in the comfort of your own home.

You can select a specific day as your "home decluttering day." It will be a day where you spend time with your kids, decluttering your home, and organizing stuff. Give your kids the chance to decide how they can help you keep things organized. Maybe one of your kids will decide on a labelling system for the boxes with the stuff. Perhaps one will be able to make DIY containers. Let your kids' imaginations run free in their organizing.

This will not only instil the habit of keeping things in order in your kids, but it will also help them develop their critical thinking and creativity in solving problems like storing stuff in a small space, lack of storage containers, recycling things, and more.

LET YOUR KIDS ORGANIZE A YARD SALE

After your decluttering activity with your kids, you can help them organize a yard sale for the excess stuff. This is especially helpful for kids aged nine and above.

You can let your kids help in placing price tags on the items. You can even let your kids help in talking to customers who will buy stuff from your yard sale. Just make sure to supervise them well. It's a sure way to teach your children the value of money as well as some incredibly basic methods for managing funds.

This will help your kids feel a sense of accomplishment. Do not forget to praise them for a job well done as well. Even if you were not able to sell everything, the fact that your kids were able to start up the yard sale should be a great learning opportunity for them already. It will help them let out their ingenuity and let them learn the ropes of business early as well.

PRAYER:

Thank you, Lord, for making us in your image. Allow us to use your gifts and imagination to make the world a better place. In the name of Jesus, Amen.

6

THE RIGHT DISCIPLINE FOR KIDS

The discipline techniques you choose will depend on the type of unacceptable behaviour that your child shows, your child's age, your child's personality, and your parenting method. It can be extremely beneficial using the following techniques.

An adult with more than one child or child care provider will agree that what succeeds with one child's parenting strategy cannot work for another. Variations in how children respond to punishment may raise a risk that their strategy is not compatible with parents.

Consequently, it is not shocking that more than one-third of parents do not believe their parenting strategies perform well, based on a survey conducted in 2007 by 2,134 parents of children aged 2 to 11.

Luckily, child psychologists have demonstrated that constructive and successful parenting methods for parents have shared foundations. Here are a few strategies to try:

CONSISTENCY IS KEY

As each person has a different parenting/caregiver style, all supervision should be apparent all the time. Help to establish clear guidelines and methods as well as expectations and incentives every day. Changes or contradictions can be challenging for youngsters, and limitations or limitations can be checked to see how far they can go for different adults. Consistency is essential for predictability in parenting. Parents become predictable to their children because their responses and outcomes are consistent. Your child will foresee how they will respond to such circumstances.

So, be consistent with your words, actions, and decisions when it comes to disciplining your child. If you are inconsistent yourself, how will you expect your child to follow the rules that you set consistently?

SEEK OUT THE 'WHY' OF MISBEHAVIOUR

If your child throws a cup and its substance spills, you would think that is unexpected, right? However, if you have time to look at the "why" of the behaviour instead of just the action itself, the child's concern (at least in this instance) might be more apparent. Whether you decide that the strokes were trapped, you might predict a result other than whether they threw it because they did not want milk for a drink. Sometimes, it could be that they were furious about something else, and that was the best way to react. Parents will always subject their child to a more acceptable action and a fair judgment by understanding their behaviour's root cause.

Disciplining your child is essential, this is something most parents are aware of. But most of the time, there is a root cause for poor behaviour that parents may neglect to examine. They may not see a way out as they feel completely in over their heads with trying to deal and manage their child's behaviour effectively. It can be incredibly overwhelming for parents. However, understand that part of the job is not just to deal with the aftereffects of poor behaviour. A big part of successful parenting is receptive to the changes in your child, especially emotionally.

So, when next you see your child acting out or doing unexpected behaviour, take time to talk to your child. Find out what is wrong instead of simply deeming it punishable. That way, you will find the "why" behind your child's behaviour and nip it in the bud, instead of allowing it to continue to fester and flourish into several other problems down the line. While parents are humans too and are not all-knowing, keeping this in mind while you discipline your children is helpful.

AVOID POWER STRUGGLES

Choose your challenges wisely – but if you have identified a fight, a parent/adult can prevail most of the time. Fix only those critical (security is still a big fight) and let other things go. But if an issue is significant, the parents should try to avoid giving in to their child, even though this is "just once." If you do, then any time this issue emerges, your child may realize that you will only change your thoughts again and groom.

So, know when to give in and when to force your way. If you see that the issue is not really that big to fuss about, then give your child some leeway. But if the problem is serious, then you absolutely cannot loosen your hold on the rules. Instead, maintain the strictness and enforce it even more.

Your child has to understand that you are the adult in the relationship and bear the responsibility of ensuring that they adopt the right habits and behaviours. For them, it means that they have to respect the boundaries that are in place between parents and children. There is a fine balance here that needs to be struck where your children understand that you love them unconditionally, but there will be consequences to poor behaviour.

EMPHASIZE AND PRAISE GOOD BEHAVIOUR

If your child's wrongdoing does not cause any harm, like tanning, whining, or other misconduct, you may opt to disregard with it. In such cases, an appropriate constructive corrective strategy may include celebrating the right actions and rewarding them with embraces, high fifths, or fun events such as a visit to the park. While it is much easier said than done to ignore a crying kid, they will ultimately learn to equate good behaviour with positive reinforcement and recognition while learning that their poor actions will not get them anything.

So, do not be stingy with your praises. If you know that your child has done well in showing good behaviour, then praise your child for it. Children thrive on praise. You don't always have to implement rewards, but simply offering kind words and praise does plenty to encourage and even inspire your children to pursue good behaviour. Remember that praises gain better results than punishment and harsh words.

KEEP YOUR COOL

Kids are fascinated by what an adult does. They are always absorbing your actions. However, they might sometimes find these activities confusing.

Talk to your child to stay calm and reassure them if they find themselves in such a state of turbulence. Teach them to remain calm and relaxed in whatever situation, even unpleasant ones. Knowing how to stay calm and cool is an essential trait to learn and must show your kids, as their immediate reaction to stressors can often be explosive. By no means are we encouraging children to bottle up their feelings. However, parents should teach their children that responding to situations calmly in order to self-regulate and manage anger is more beneficial. Forgoing this can bring about several problems for your child's future, as they are met with increasingly challenging social situations. It can cause a lot of damage and be a deterrent for future relationships your child will have with other people.

As you instil being calm to your kids, you must also exhibit this trait, especially in front of them. Remember that children learn better when they have someone to refer to the trait. So, if you want your children to grow calm and know how to keep their cool, you better do it yourself first.

SEEK OUT DISCIPLINE SUPPORTERS

Whenever someone else watches your child, make sure that you express your discipline method and urge the guardian to follow a similar approach. Likewise, if you do not believe in a specific solution, please tell a babysitter or an early childhood teacher of this too. Take the opportunity to inquire about their training techniques to look for a potential daycare or nursery. Parents will find that the findings become more successful if they align their methodology to childcare approaches. The explanation may be that children respond to behavioural tactics used by their peers.

When someone else takes the helm of disciplining your child, even for just a day, you must make sure that whoever it is, they know your discipline style. For example, if you do not allow your child to eat ice cream past 9: 00 PM, then the baby sitter should adhere to this rule as well, no matter how your child begs them to consider.

EDUCATE YOURSELF ON PARENTING AND DISCIPLINE STYLES

There are various varieties of parental methods and disciplinary techniques. Training in different ideas will allow you to be more knowledgeable and regulated when deciding how to respond to your child's circumstance. If you chose optimistic, boundary-based, gentle, or other styles, it is essential to understand what every style is and choose what best suits your culture.

You need to brush up on these parenting styles so you could shape a style of your own that will best fit your children. Try to listen to how other parents deal with their children and pick up what you think will work for you. Doing research and reading parenting books are also great resources where you can learn.

While there can be so many tips and tricks out there that parents swear by, finding one that suits yourself and your child can be a gargantuan task. But part of the process is trusting yourself to know what comes naturally to you as ultimately, you know yourself and your children the best.

HEALTHY DISCIPLINE STRATEGIES THAT WORK

The AAP recommends positive discipline strategies, which effectively educate and prevent children from harming their actions while promoting healthy growth. This includes the following:

- Show and tell. Teach kids right from wrong with steady words and deeds. You want to see model patterns in your children.
- Set restrictions. Have consistent and straightforward guidelines that your kids should obey. Make sure to clarify these laws in age-appropriate terminology.
- Give results. Explain the consequences politely and firmly if they do not act. For example, remind him/her that you are going to put it away for the rest of the day if he/she does not choose his/her toys. Be able to step up directly. Do not give in for a few minutes by handing them up. But please, never take anything your child wants like a meal away.
- Hear them out. Listening is important. It is important. Enable your child to complete the story before solving the dilemma. Look for occasions when wrongdoing has a trend. Speak about this with your kid; do not just offer implications.
- Give them your attention. Attention is an essential weapon for successful discipline to improve positive conduct and deter others. Note, both children want the love of their parents.
- Catch them good. Children deserve to know when they are doing something wrong and when they are doing something right. Note positive conduct and

show it, enjoy the performance and successful attempts. Be descriptive ("wow, you've done a nice job putting the toy away!"). Be precise.

- Know when not to speak. If your kid does not do anything dangerous and thinks about acceptable behaviour, avoiding negative behaviour may be a successful way to prevent it. Misconduct will also show children the normal results of their behaviour.

- Be prepared for difficulties. Hop for whenever your child has problems acting. Prepare them and the way you expect them to behave.

- Bad actions reverse. Often children's misbehaviour is usually due to whether they are lonely or because they do not know anything better. Find out what your child would love to do and set them right in.

- Call timeout. A pause can be beneficial if a particular law is violated. This method works well to warn kids if they do not quit, warning them of what they have DONE wrong. You should only say "go back and forth whenever you are comfortable and in charge," which can help the child develop and improve self-management skills, which works well for the elderly and teenagers.

RESPONDING TO TANTRUMS

When a child is tired, starving, irritated, or frustrated, tantrums usually result. Maybe your child would keep her fists clenched, close her eyes, and scream. He may kick, throw himself to the floor, and create a scene around it.

Make efforts to prevent tantrums from happening. Ensure your child gets enough sleep. Do not take them out when they are tired or hungry. If you must do, bring along healthy kids, food, toys, or books to keep your child engaged throughout the outing.

Why are tantrums so common at this age?

- Kids are curious and explore all they can to find answers to what amuses them.
- Children are faced with new emotions and a natural response to convey some of these complicated emotions and display their discomfort is through a tantrum.
- Because they might not express themselves adequately, they might turn out to become angry.
- When children are hungry or frustrated, they often react with unpleasant emotions or behaviour.

Keep in mind that tantrums are normal among kids. So, leave them to experience this if they are not hurting themselves or someone else.

What can you do as a parent?

Try Distraction: distracting your child from their interest in something else works in your response to a tantrum as a parent.

TIPS FOR APPLYING CONSEQUENCES

- Apply consequences almost immediately.
- Avoid getting into arguments with your kids during the correction process.
- Make the consequences short. For instance, the timeout should be for just a minute to a maximum of 5 minutes (depending on the child's age).
- Be serious when you correct the kids but do not yell at them.
- Explain to them why they are being punished for their behaviour. They should be able to explain back to you why they acted in such a way and that it is wrong.
- Always follow consequences with love and care.

BELOW ARE SOME EXCERPTS.

- Avoid nagging and making threats without consequences. The latter may even encourage undesired behaviour.
- Apply rules steadily.
- Ignore irrelevant behaviour such as swinging legs while sitting.
- Set achievable limits, maybe every week.
- State acceptable and right behaviour that is workable.
- Prioritize rules. Giving safety top priority, then to correct actions that damage individuals and property, and then to conducts such as temper tantrums and disruption. You may focus on two or three rules for a start.
- Accept mistakes bound to their age limit. For instance, they were accidentally spilling water on the floor.
- Understand their temperament and raise them accordingly.

PROBLEM HANDLING FOR CHILDREN

If your kid cannot find his math homework or forgets his lunch, the secret to helping him navigate his life is strong problem-solving skills.

In a 2010 report released in Behaviour Science and Treatment, the risk of depression and suicide was greater for children lacking problem-solving skills.

The researchers have found that teaching a child problem-solving skill would enhance their emotional health.

You will continue to teach simple problems during preschool, which will help your child develop their high school skills and beyond.

REASONS KIDS NEED PROBLEM-SOLVING MINDSET

Children face a host of challenges every day, from school issues to athletics challenges. However, a few of them have a method to fix these issues.

Instead of investing their resources into fixing the problem, they will spend time ignoring the problem. Therefore, so many children fall behind in school or why they fail to keep friends.

Some children who lack the desire to overcome difficulties do not understand their decisions. A child can strike a peer who cuts in line in front of him because he does not know what else he should do.

If he is tinkered, he may go out of class because he cannot think of any better way to stop it. These impulsive actions will, in the long-term, cause much greater problems.

TEACH KIDS HOW TO EVALUATE THE PROBLEM

Children who feel confused or helpless will sometimes not want to fix a dilemma. However, they will be secure in their ability to solve a crisis when you give them a simple method or guide to solve problems.

Here are the steps to solve the problem:

- Define the problem. Simply mentioning the issue will make a significant impact on children who feel lost. Support your child to state the case, for example, "You have no one with whom to play in recess," or "You do not know whether you can take advanced math's."
- Create five potential alternatives at least It should be emphasized that not all proposals ought to be successful at concepts (at least not at present). Support your child to develop strategies if they fail to generate ideas. Such a dumb explanation or a far-fetched idea is conceivable. The key is to make him see that he can discover several different alternative options with a little imagination.
- Identify the benefits and disadvantages of each approach. Help your child consider potential positive and negative outcomes with any possible solution it has found.
- Choose a solution. After the future good and bad effects have been measured, motivate your child to find a solution.
- Try it out. Find a solution to see what is going on. If it does not fit, he/she can still find a different approach in phase 2 of the list he/she created.

There are unavoidable bumps, potholes, and unsafe zones in addition to all the valuable moments and memorable memories.

It may feel a little like a ride down a bumpy path to help your child solve problems, encounter dead-end after dead-end, and lose sight of the target.

You want your child to feel like you are working together to fix issues and not just lecturing and wiping them up!

TIPS FOR PROBLEM-SOLVING WITH YOUR CHILD

Here, then, are some tips to manoeuvre through the problem-solving minefield with your child:

1. Try not to play the role of "Mr./Mrs. Fix-It".

Sometimes, children are disappointed by a solution that is not correct now with their unique situation. So, give your child autonomy and a chance to work things out for him/herself. Remember that experiencing the process of decision-making and looking for solutions for problems can be a better lesson for your child, rather than fixing the problem yourself and telling your child about it.

2. Help them to find their answers and solutions.

As parents, you want to do all right, of course, but in the end, you want to encourage problem-solving in your girl/boy.

By encouraging your child to find his/her ideas and responses, you motivate the child to feel empowered and deal with the skills. As your child feels empowered to solve the issues, he/she is dealing with, and it will breed even more sense of achievement. It is a cycle. So, you must be a pillar of support and be a guide for your child as he/she tries to solve problems.

3. Teach your child how they can "survive" difficult or unpleasant feelings.

Although they may not feel confident about frustration, rage, sadness, and remorse yet, your child needs to learn to control these emotions until they eventually occur. Explain to your child that feeling these emotions are normal and that they should not feel afraid of it. Instead, encourage your child to take control of these emotions and "survive." This helps to create strength to cope. You need to emphasize that once your child takes charge of these emotions, it will be easier for them to think more logically despite being angry.

4. Try to keep the focus on your child and not you.

You may feel hesitant to offer your personal experience with a similar issue. Instead, just listen and offer your support if your kids ask for it. Sometimes your child simply needs a shoulder to cry on, or sometimes they may approach you to help them out of a situation. Anticipating their needs or even verbalizing what they need in the current situation is an excellent strategy to make sure you keep the focus on your child and help them feel seen during difficult times.

Kids sometimes do not like it when their parents meddle with their personal affairs. So, if the issue is not pressing enough to cause concern, let your child handle it. Then, when your child seeks you for help, then that is the time that you act.

5. Children feel better when they feel understood.

Children will accept more than merely being offered a solution. Remember that kids can think on their own as well. Sometimes kids would rather have you not provide a solution for their problem but understand them and know where they are coming from, rather than you offering a solution. It's helpful to try and relate to your child's situation and recall how you might have felt at that age. Recall yourself ever facing the same situation or consider how you might have reacted. Be open and honest with your children when you try to understand them. Sometimes you may not even know how they feel but being able to empathize and show compassion is so important.

Do not alienate yourself from the problem, but not be too meddlesome either. Listen to what your child has to say. Put yourself on his/her shoe and view the situation from their perspective. That will be a much better "solution" you can offer to your child.

6. Timing is everything.

After a long day at school, children need to rest and refresh their batteries.

There is no right time to have deep conversations and a conversation that addresses problems (this is also the moment that monosyllables respond to parents!).

Instead, why not schedule a specific time at home for a few minutes of chat? Scheduling a type gives your children a chance to prepare themselves, and the same goes for parents as well.

This could be before bed, after they cool down, or maybe after "working time" or "meetings." It is smart to try to relax them — maybe even over tea/coffee, hot cocoa, or a sweet treat! Get your children comfortable and let them know that they can divulge anything they want without fear of repercussions. This is a time for them to express what has been weighing heavily on them, or negatively impacting them. It may even only be a chance to share the positive things that have been affecting their lives. Whatever they choose to talk about, it is your chance to get a deeper understanding of your child.

When you approach your children to engage in a heart-to-heart conservation, you need them in a time where they are not busy, relaxed, and ready to open. Do not suddenly spring a conversation with them on deep or heavy topics when they are not mentally prepared or anticipating it. But once you do start with the deep conversations, you can make this a routine either daily or weekly. It is even better if you have a scheduled daily "check-up" talk and a weekly "deep" talk.

7. Encourage your child to think, plan, and reassess before acting.

You help them learn an essential life skill by showing them that resolving problems is not an immediate answer but a continuous process. You must make your child understand that solving real-life problems is not like problems solved at school, where you only must perform a certain step, and you will already get the answer. Emphasize to your child that problems in life are more complicated than they think. They themselves are a process, and that as you look for ways to solve them, you need to think, plan, and reassess things before you can find the best solution.

Furthermore, this can encourage children to be more result-oriented where they begin assessing their abilities through their performance, rather than the achievement at the end. This is a great way to get your kids to strive to perform better and look at themselves critically as they follow through with their plans.

You can also let your child read newspapers or chat with friends for experience in sharing their opinions and listening to other people. They will also benefit from picking up views in a newspaper or chatting to others as they learn about the diversity that exists around us.

8. Asking for help is a sign of strength, not weakness.

Kids sometimes think that asking for help from others, especially their parents, is a sign of weakness. You need to make your kids understand that asking for help is not a weakness but a strength. Remember this and instil this in the mind of your kid before your kid accepts it!

But you also must emphasize that asking for help every time is also not a good practice. Your kid should know when to ask for help and when to rely on him/herself. With this, you will be able to develop a sense of independence in your child and a sense of confidence in their abilities to solve problems on their own or seek help from others.

9. Applaud your child's strengths and focus on positive outcomes.

Your child needs positive reinforcement and not just constant reminders and notifications of their misdemeanours. This is where parents have to find a suitable medium between disciplining their children and focusing on their good behaviour. When you notice that your child has done something right or accomplished a task, you must acknowledge that.

Tell them you are proud of their contributions to coping with stringent circumstances. You will soon notice that your child will take an even more active role in helping you.

Be specific and descriptive with your words as effusive positive words can come off disingenuous or insincere as the more general it is, the less likely it is to be relevant to your child. ("I'm an angel for sharing my toys? What about not doing homework last night?") Children can sometimes perceive the disingenuous praise and instead use it to reflect on their behaviour and consider how they acted contrary to the praise when you use sweeping terms for praise.

10. Encourage your child to have a support network.

Emphasize to your child that being alone in dealing with problems is not good. You need to make your child understand the importance of keeping the right friends and being open to family. Bottling up feelings and pent up anger can lead to disastrous results.

As a parent, you can provide a safe space for your kids to share their feelings and express anything that has had a negative impact on their mental health. Be a non-judgmental listener and provide support when they need it. Support comes in plenty of forms, sometimes it means being a shoulder to cry on, or sometimes it means being more proactive and providing the solution outright to them. Regardless of the issue and its scope, being present for your child is crucial for their development.

At the same time, your child can also have other people involved in their support system to ground them and help them navigate through life. This can be anyone your child will feel comfortable to approach and divulge their feelings with. Many adults, family members and peers can become involved in their support system. As long as your child does not feel alone or like an outcast or afterthought, you are already taking steps in the right direction.

Remember that every parenting (family) journey is different, and a destination is reached in several ways. So, do not limit your options to yourself. If others can help your child, then include them. As much as parents cling onto the idea of their children being dependent on them for a very long time, they eventually have to let go of this notion and allow their children to peacefully make their own social connections and build trust with other people who may enter into their lives.

PRACTICE SOLVING PROBLEMS

Do not rush to fix your child's issues for him if difficulties occur. Help him go over the problem-solving phase instead. Provide advice when he needs support, but empower him to fix things himself.

If he cannot find a way, move in to make him learn of available options. The key is to avoid telling him what to do immediately because you want your children to be able to process a new situation and figure out the best course of action independently.

You need to serve as the guide for your child and not the problem-solver. If you solve every single problem your child experiences, how will they learn and grow? So, give your child the chance to think on their own and look for solutions to their problems. But welcome them as well if they take the initiative to ask for your help. Encourage different ways to approach solutions and be a source for your child to bounce their ideas off of. You can still provide advice for your child, but encourage them to voice what they think and what they feel compelled to do in the situation.

Using a problem-solving strategy when you experience behavioural problems:

Solving problems that involve your child can be difficult. That is why you need to have a solid strategy on how to deal with them.

For example, you can sit down with your child and say, "It was challenging to get your homework done lately. Let us solve it together."

You will also have to deal with their misbehaviour, and the same thing applies. You need to be sure that you have invested in finding a solution so that your kids can do better next time.

8

HOW TO RAISE YOUR TYPE OF CHILD

One of the mistakes that parents often commit when raising their children is that they do not consider what type of child they have. A disciplinary action that is effective for one child may not be as effective for another child.

That is because children varied in their personalities and thought processes. Some children are more sensitive than others. Some are more difficult than others. In comparison, some are clever and need less supervision.

If you want to raise your child well, you need to consider the things that make your child unique: their learning styles, their habits, their personality, etc. No two children are the same, and as such, no single parenting method is going to apply effectively to every child. Your children do not fall into a category but instead may inhibit certain characteristics. Ultimately, children are a mix of all of the following "types". Some children may be more emotional than others. The same be said about stubborn or strong-willed children. Finding the right parenting style is part of the journey of parenthood that must be faced. Mothers and fathers can then apply the necessary disciplinary actions according to their child's needs.

RAISING AN EMOTIONAL CHILD

One of the main problems with emotional children is that they do not have a full grasp of their emotions. They can cry for the littlest things. It does not also help that many parents have negative reactions when they see their child crying, especially in public. This should not be. If your child is emotional, here are some tips that you can apply:

Crying is not necessarily a weakness. It is usual for children to cry, but some parents become embarrassed if their child cries in public. For example, a father may see his child crying over fallen ice cream. The father cringes from the scene and immediately scolds the child or takes the child away. The same thing may happen for a mother who sees her daughter crying because she lost.

If your child is emotional, it does not mean that your child is weak. They simply do not have control of their emotions yet. That is why, as parents, it is your role to help your child recognize their emotions and understand how to control them.

Put a name on the emotion. Sometimes a child may cry but may not fully understand why they are really crying. You must put a name on the emotion they are feeling. For example, you can say, "You are crying because you are sad that you lost." You can name your emotions as well so that the child can relate to how you feel. You can say, "I am sad that you did not do your homework today."

You can drill on this by watching movies or reading books and asking the child how the characters are feeling. It will help them associate the names of emotions with how they look and feel.

Differentiate feelings and behaviour. You must tell your child that they can feel all those emotions, but they can decide on how to respond to those emotions. You need to emphasize that there are certain behaviours more appropriate for a certain emotion. For example, you can say, "It is okay to be angry, but you cannot hit anyone because of it." Or, "It is okay to cry, but you cannot throw a tantrum."

Discipline the behaviour, not the emotions. Inform your child that whatever emotions they feel, it is normal, but once they behave inappropriate in response to those emotions, then there are consequences. For example, you can say, "I will be taking your toys for a day because you were screaming when you cried, and it is not a good behaviour." Allow your children to express their emotions in an appropriate way, rather than encouraging them to suppress them.

Do not minimize a child's emotions. One mistake that many parents commit is underestimating their child's feelings. For example, some parents will tell their child to stop crying because the problem is not a crying matter. This is wrong. You need to validate what and how your child feels so they can better understand. For example, you can say, "You are mad because I did not buy you ice cream. I also get mad when I do not get what I want too. But you should not cry about it because there is still next time, or another day called tomorrow."

Teach emotion regulation. You need to teach your child how they can regulate and manage their emotions and keep them under control. Here are some skills you can teach:

1. Take a quiet moment to process their emotions.
2. Try some deep breathing exercising to regulate your heart and breathing.
3. Count from 1 to 10.
4. Closing their eyes and relax.
5. Create a kit to cheer up.
6. Do a hobby to boost mood.

RAISING AN EMPATHIC CHILD

Empathic kids understand the feelings of others and know how to deal with their own emotions and the emotions of others. If you want your child to develop empathy, then here are some tips:

Help your child understand their own feelings. Empathic people understand the feelings of others because they have a full understanding of their feelings. You need to help your child make sense of their emotions first. Explain what positive and negative emotions are and what your child can do in response to them.

Do not hide the truth. Some parents shield their children from the harsh realities of the world, which downgrades the importance of these realities. This can give the wrong impression to the child that these issues do not matter. Talk about these issues (e.g., bullying, school shootings, allergies, the effect of coronavirus, global crisis) with your child and make them understand their importance. Even if they do not thoroughly understand them yet, at least they will have an idea.

A demonstration is a good option. If you want your child to be empathic, then you have to be empathic yourself. Stay calm in stressful situations. Process your emotions first before reacting immediately. Model this to your child.

Take action and show kindness. Actions speak louder than words. Model kind behaviour if you want your children to do the same. Take a moment of your day to slow down and show kindness to others. Any small act will do as ultimately, and your children are always observing how you treat others and will absorb the same behaviours and habits. Help an elderly cross the street. Help the neighbour with a chore. How you display your capacity for compassion can really leave a mark on your children. These are little things that when you show your child, they will still realize the importance of being kind.

RAISING A STRONG-WILLED CHILD

Raising a strong-willed child is probably one of the greatest challenges of a parent. That is because, unlike other children, strong-willed children tend to be more stubborn and courageous enough to defy their parents, especially if they have their own viewpoints against a particular matter. Therefore, most parents who have strong-willed children end up in a power-struggle against their own kids. If you are experiencing the same problem with your child, then here are some tips you can follow:

Teach through experience. Strong-willed children learn best through experience. That is why they do not easily believe what you say when they do not experience it themselves. For example, when you tell your child not to touch the stove because it is hot, they will confirm if it is hot before they believe you. Use that to your advantage. When you discipline your child, it is best if they experience the effect first, unless there is a risk for serious injury.

Give them independence. It is better if you give your child to be independent. Instead of nagging them to do things, give them reminders instead. For example, instead of telling a child to do their homework and not play, you can say, "Before playing, what do you need to do?" This way, you are not directly telling them what to do but reminding them by asking the question.

Do not give orders. Like giving them independence, give your child choices instead of orders. It affords them the autonomy that they deserve. For example, you need to ask your child to do some chores, but they are playing. You can say, "You need to pause your playing for a moment and help me with the trash. Do you want to help me now and still have a chance to play before bed? Or do you want to continue playing and help me with the trash later. But it's going to be too dark outside later on." Being a figure of authority in a child's life does not mean that every order you demand should be met.

Implement routines. To avoid having to constantly wrestle power from your child and being the bad guy for forcing them, you need to set up a routine and ground rules. Children thrive on a routine because it sets their days up in an organized way so that they know what to expect and aren't overwhelmed by the possibilities. You must make sure that your child agrees to them as well. That way, when your child commits something that breaks the rules, you must remind them that they agreed to the routine and the rules beforehand, including the consequences.

Listen to what your child has to say. Your child has their own views and opinions on things. You must listen to what they say. Even when you know they are wrong, give them a chance to share why they think are right. By listening carefully, will you understand why your child is opposing you or acting in a certain way? This will also help you see the issue from their point of view.

Respect your children. As you expect your children to respect you, the same goes vice versa. Children are human beings and deserve respect as they navigate through life. Since your child has strong views on things, you must respect that. Make them understand your views by talking about it to them. In the same way, discuss their views with them as well. This will help both you and your child, where each of you is coming from regarding the problem. These are opportune moments to teach your child that people are always going to have a different perspective, and not everyone will agree with them.

FINAL THOUGHTS

Raising a child is never easy. Parenthood is not something that is taught in schools, and the best way to truly get a good grasp on being a parent is through experience. You learn as you go along and experience what it is like to raise a child. However, one thing that you should really put effort into understanding is how to raise your child is their nature. Do not lump your child together with your friend's child. All children are incredibly different and unique from each other and have been shaped by different things in their lives. Your disciplinary methods must match the type of child that you have. Only then will you be able to observe positive changes in their behaviours.

LEAVE A REVIEW!

After reading this book, please feel free to leave a review based on your findings and how useful the guide was to you. I would be incredibly thankful if you could take 60 seconds to write a brief review on Amazon, even if it's just a few sentences!

CONCLUSION

Discipline is about behaviour modification, not about punishing kids. Discipline encourages kids to develop self-discipline and helps them become adults who are mentally and socially mature. Many efficient approaches can help parents teach their children and direct them, and certain types of discipline will remain controversial.

As you try to instil good habits and good behaviour within your children, parents will sometimes come across moments of anxiety as they question their capabilities and their methods. This is something that parents around the world have experienced for generations. Being a good parent is a Herculean task, but by no means is it impossible. Having faith and trusting in your own capabilities to love and nourish your children comes first to being a good parent. From this vantage point, as you discipline your children and walk them through life, you will be bound to make mistakes but know that children are resilient in their own way. Be vulnerable with your children and respect them so that you realize when it is time to apologize to them.

Always remember that there is no one right way to train a child. Do your best, trust God to help you, and enjoy the company of the little ones in your life.

REFERENCES

Tips for Parents: Teaching Discipline to Your Children. Retrieved from https://preventchildabuse.org/resource/tips-for-parents-teaching-discipline-to-your-children/

School Administrator's Top 10 Discipline Tips All Parents Should Know. Retrieved from http://www.parent-institute.com/reports-for-delivery/10-Discipline-Tips-Report.pdf

Discipline (0 – 12 years). Retrieved from https://www.education.sa.gov.au/sites/default/files/parentingsa/peg2.pdf?v=1489727260

Discipline in the Early Years. Retrieved from http://learnatcstreet.org/data/documents/Child-Discipline.pdf

How to Discipline Toddlers by Rachel Ehmke. Retrieved from https://childmind.org/article/how-discipline-toddlers/

Three Principles to Improve Outcomes for Children and Families by Center on the Developing Child, Harvard University. Retrieved from https://developingchild.harvard.edu/resources/three-early-childhood-development-principles-improve-child-family-outcomes/

Effective discipline for children. (2004). *Pediatrics & child health*, *9*(1), 37–50. Retrieved from https://doi.org/10.1093/pch/9.1.37

Discipline and Guiding Behaviour**: Babies and Children.** Retrieved from https://raisingchildren.net.au/toddlers/behaviour/discipline/discipline-strategies#choosing-an-approach-to-discipline-nav-title

Positive Discipline: A Guide for Parents. Retrieved from http://pcit-toddlers.org/resources/umn-positive-discipline-a-guide-for-parents.pdf

Great Habits for Kids to Have Early in Life. Retrieved from https://afgfamily.com/blog/news/8-great-habits-for-kids-to-have-early-in-life/

https://parenting.firstcry.com/articles/12-habits-of-parents-who-are-raising-successful-children/

An age-by-age guide to disciplining your kid. Retrieved from https://www.todaysparent.com/kids/preschool/disciplining-children-age-by-age-guide/

Parents, Kids, and Discipline. Retrieved from https://www.webmd.com/parenting/guide/discipline-tactics

God made you be creative. Retrieved from https://douglastalks.com/god-made-you-to-be-creative-a-lesson-about-creativity-for-kids/

Ways to Boost Child's Creative Thinking. Retrieved from https://ezplaytoys.com/blogs/blog/creativity-for-kids-15-ways-to-boost-childs-creative-thinking

How to Help an Overly Emotional Child Cope with Their Feelings. Retrieved from https://www.verywellfamily.com/how-to-help-an-overly-emotional-child-4157594

4 Ways to Raise an Empathic Child. Retrieved from https://www.positiveparentingsolutions.com/parenting/4-ways-to-raise-an-empathy-rich-child

The strong-willed child: 11 ways to turn power struggles into cooperation. Retrieved from https://

www.mother.ly/child/11-tips-for-parenting-your-strong-willed-child/5-avoid-power-struggles-by-using-routines-and-rules

Like us on https://www.facebook.com/tcecpublishing/

http://www.thechildrenseducationcentre.co.uk/specialoffer

HEALTHY HABITS FOR KIDS

POSITIVE PARENTING TIPS FOR FUN KIDS
EXERCISES, HEALTHY SNACKS AND
IMPROVED KIDS NUTRITION

INTRODUCTION

Children are incredibly perceptive beings who soak up their surroundings like proverbial sponges. They are like a blank slate, and as they age with the guidance of their parents, each stage of their life is marked by new experiences and emotions. The most natural thing for them to do is to imitate the people closest to them, and when they are young, parents and siblings become their primary role models. Your kids are likely to adopt the same habits as yours; from the way you eat and sleep to the little things in your personality that you might not be aware of that your children end up mimicking, whether intentional or not.

As a result, parents can be overly cautious when it comes to raising their kids for fear of making mistakes and teaching your children the wrong things. But parenting is a massive learning curve for any new mother or father. For many, understanding that it is a journey that will be filled with success and failures is crucial. Turning to guides such as this one is a great way to get you started on the right foot in your journey. It provides a foundational basis to tackle some of the biggest questions and concerns parents have when it comes to their kids' health and wellbeing.

As a parent, you are the biggest influence on your children's health habits. This is possibly the most significant point to take from this book. Understand that your children are continually surveilling you and everything that you do or say will be copied at some point, which is why it is so crucial to adopt reasonable, practical habits that prioritize your mental and physical health for your children to feel motivated to do the same. You have a significant impact on the environment where your kids grow up, and you are responsible for the way they eat their meals, the types of food they eat, and so much more. For instance, neophobia, a persistent fear for anything new, can often blossom in children who have not been recipients of good parenting and the presence of positive role models while growing up. Kids are more likely to try new foods if they have noticed someone else eating them. Moreover, when parents take a bite of their kid's food and show signs of delight, kids are more likely to crave that food.

Research shows that parenting beliefs or behaviours affect development in infancy employing different pathways. A parent-provided experience might influence the infant at a particular point in time in a specific way, and the consequence is lasting on the infant, independent of later parenting and of any other contribution of the infant. Theoreticians and researchers have long supposed that the child's earliest experiences affect the course of later development.

Keep in mind that habits are difficult to break. So, the faster we develop good, safe habits that are consistent in life, the easier it is to stay and keep these habits throughout life. Also, it's easier to avoid bad habits when healthy habits are in place since the early, developmental stages.

For children, parents represent a model of behaviour and attitudes, and children often look to their parents to navigate their way through life. Parents serve as a reference point for their children as someone to guide them when they find themselves in trouble, and kids adopt this tradition early in their lives. As they grow up, children mimic their parents' behaviour and actions as they experience new things and respond to new situations. Therefore, it is necessary to teach children how to distinguish between good and bad habits and choose the right ones.

Being a parent is a beautiful thing; however, it's not always easy. It brings its myriad of challenges and forces the parent to look beyond their well-being to wholly bear the responsibility of caring for another person. Hopefully, the information in this book will show you how you can guide, nurture, and improve your kids and their overall health habits as a parent.

After reading this book, please feel free to leave a review based on your findings and how useful the guide was to you. I would be incredibly thankful if you could take 60 seconds to write a brief review on Amazon, even if it's just a few sentences!

WAYS TO ENCOURAGE YOUR CHILD TO BE PHYSICALLY DYNAMIC

We all know that being physically dynamic is vital for our wellbeing, but it can be hard to find the time with our busy schedules. Our children face the same challenges. They have education, homework and plenty of extracurricular work that is continually being challenged by the temptations of TV, video games, the Internet and social media, whether they have their mobile iPod or iPad. Today, on average, children spend over 30 hours per week watching television. Children need moderate to intense physical activity each day for at least 60 minutes, yet this continues to be neglected by most children.

Here are a few ways to inspire your children to become more active:

Be a good role model

While many parents live according to the phrase, "do as I say, not what I do," we as parents have a more decisive influence on children by influencing their healthy behaviour. Ensure you make time to exercise in your regular or weekly schedule and let your children see you doing this. National guidelines suggest that adults should obtain at least 150 minutes of physical exercise a week and aim to do something productive for at least 30 minutes, five days a week. If you are active, there's a higher tendency of engaging your children also to be involved.

Motivate them to join sports or other organized physical activities

Motivate your children to try various sports such as football, basketball, baseball, or the track team. If you're not an athlete, you can enjoy dance or cheerleading. Doing something with like-minded children can help your child remain involved and encourage their level of operation. Joining a team will also open your children up to new opportunities to engage with the social dimensions of the team's experience. This not only encourages fitness, but it also fosters social skills that are crucial to a child's development.

Be creative about finding a free physical activity

Organized sports can be costly with all the facilities and expenses so it might not always be practical. However, your children can still get the right amount of physical activity without it. The solution is to be more proactive in finding creative ways to get your kids involved in physical activity. There are quite a few options that you do not need to break the bank and can be done reasonably quickly within your household if your work program does not allow you to get your child to daily baseball practices and games.

Here are several schemes:

- Spend some time with your children at your local park or playground.
- Play some of your child's favourite music and get them dancing.
- When you work around the house, allow your children to play outside with their siblings or neighbours when the weather is good. Or go out and play catch or tag.
- Let your child play energetic games in the house on rainy days. A little noise is not going to harm you.
- Do workouts together as a family in your home.
- Reap double the advantages by having your children do chores; vacuuming and staining or

raking the leaves benefits you and can also be a good workout.

Any physical activity is better than zero, so keep your children going.

Keep electronic temptations at a minimum

Today, most households have several TVs in the house and combine appliances with video game systems and mobile telephones, making it impossible to fight temptations of spending hours at a time glued to a screen. However, you and your kids should encourage electronic-free time to do fun, active things together that engages everyone's interests. Do not let your children have a TV or laptop in their room and keep tabs electronic on their electronic usage. As stated by the American Academy of Pediatrics, children's average should not exceed one to two hours a day. Set an example by modelling this behaviour, as adults can also fall into the same trap of focusing on their phones rather than what is going on around them. While electronic devices can be a great way to distract your children for some time, it can also be to their detriment.

Help your child find his/her passion

If they are excited about it, your child will be more likely to continue an activity. Your goal as a parent is to support them and help them find what they will thrive in. Whether it is baseball, dance, or walking, any physical activity is pleasant. The most important thing is that they are excited and enthusiastic about doing it.

Emphasize safety in all they do

Ensure you don't overdo physical activity or exercise and speak to your doctor about any protection you should take and any mark or symptoms you should be vigilant of. Recall that the benefits of physical activity are far greater than the risk of injury.

Make exercise a priority

The essential thing to note is that a healthy body and mind needs a balanced diet and daily exercise. One will not be as successful without the other. Teach your kids what they should eat and how much they should move their bodies, and the faster they get started, the better. Bear in mind that it is never too late to start cultivating healthy behaviours from an early age. So, regardless of your children's age now, get them going today.

Many parents struggle to find an activity that would interest their child and relinquish their dependence on passing the time by watching TV. A great way to combat this is by working with your child's teachers and being aware of where your child is excelling in school. In one instance, a parent found out that their child had excelled in the dance unit in their physical education class and ended up enrolling their child in professional dance lessons which have since led to several benefits. Not only has their cardiovascular health improved by leaps and bounds, but the child has also gained a new cohort of friends from their dance class, who serve as another support system outside of school and their home. Part of your journey as the parent is to understand your child and help them navigate through life. Fostering their talents more often than not lead to a significant number of benefits that you may not even be expecting. The key here is to be proactive and find ways to engage your child.

7 STYLES TO HELP GET YOUR KIDS TO BRUSH REGULARLY

You know how necessary it is for your children to clean their teeth daily, but it often feels like pushing a mountain. It is obvious that your child will fight you when it comes to doing something good for them, like bathing or eating their vegetables. And it's no different to brushing their teeth. It may not look like a big deal when your child is incredibly fussy, but it may be a slippery slope that can lead to bad oral habits and poor oral hygiene for a lifetime. Dentists have seen an increase in the number of cavities in preschool-age children in recent years, which is significant and must be tackled.

The easiest way to avoid dental problems early in their life is by them starting to brush their teeth as early as possible.

Here are a few ways to engage your children to brush regularly without losing their cool in the process:

Model good behaviour

Kids are like sponges. They watch your actions and want to be like you. When they see you brushing your teeth and flossing twice a day, they automatically feel compelled to mirror the same behaviour that you also encourage to be good. They will see how vital it is to have a clean mouth. Make them stand at the sink as you brush your teeth so that they can see the right motions through the process. Even brush your teeth together. Let them choose their fun toothbrush and toothpaste flavour so that they are excited to brush their teeth every day.

If you know that your dental habits are lax, you need to deal with them as soon as possible because your child is more likely to develop good habits as you practice good habits.

Explain why it is so important

Some children need an explanation when they attempt to comprehend the world around them. If your child is curious, take the time to break down and explain why regular teeth brushing is so important. Explain the cavities and plaque and what can happen over time to your teeth. Give them a sense of control of their bodies, so they know they are making the right decision. You don't want to frighten them but give them ample details to make them take it seriously.

Do a little experiment.

If your child wants more help and wants experimental tests, ask your dentist or pharmacist for a dissolving agent that can highlight the plaque on your child's teeth. All your child has to do is to chew the tablet, and when they open their mouth, their teeth will appear pink with plaque. You can't deny what happens when you don't clean it correctly when you look at it in the mirror.

Make brushing fun

Children want to have fun and don't want to sit and take the time to do something that takes them away from the more exciting thing at their disposal. Who would brush their teeth if they could play outside? The easiest way to combat this is to have fun with brushing. One suggestion that pediatric dentists sometimes make is that they sing "The wheels go around" as they brush their teeth. It is more enjoyable, and it makes them follow the correct brushing method; instead of brushing back and forth, actually doing round strokes.

You may even have a contest bubbling your teeth together. You may also persuade your kid to brush their teeth using a favourite toy like a teddy or baby doll.

Help them keep time

Children and patience do not go together, and they naturally want to hurry with their teeth brushing to have fun, so we need to help them keep their time better, so they can brush their teeth for the prescribed 2 minutes. Simple methods include singing a song while brushing and reminding them they can't stop until the song is over. Or make them count the time or give them an egg timer after two minutes.

Set aside proper time for it

You don't have enough time for proper brushing if you run consistently late in the morning to get them out of bed while they are still sleepy. A tired child coupled with a stressed-out parent means that the brushing of teeth is at most a reluctant slap affair. You can set the time for when you are not in a hurry and when your child is aware, this will make the whole process far less difficult for you and your child.

Be their cheering squad.

Finally, praise your children when they follow through with the correct way to brush their teeth. They will not only feel good about the efforts that they have put in, but it will also stress how critical following their everyday routine is.

But don't be afraid to ask your dentist for advice if your child tries to battle with you with acceptable brushing practices.

Often the external encouragement from another authority figure is what a child needs to take things seriously. It's a relentless battle, even with the team strategy. But as the parent, don't give up. Although it may be tempting to let your child's behaviour slide, it can have adverse effects. It is vital for your child's long-term wellbeing to now turn it into a daily routine. Cavities and gum disease can lead to costly and painful dental problems for a lifetime. It is not always easy to get your kids to brush their teeth every morning and evening, but even so, it must be done regularly.

3

WHAT IS HEALTHY EATING?

Parents are responsible for the early education of their kids. You have the opportunity to teach your kids to appreciate nutritious foods by leveraging creative children's activities about healthy eating.

Learning about foods does not have to be a dreaded thing. Children can have fun while learning about foods – basically sweet foods and other food groups.

You can create amazing chances for learning about healthy food in several ways, including using games, songs, crafts, dance, and more. For instance, instead of playing the classic game "Candyland", you can make up a life-size "Veggieland" game board.

With having some extra patience, creativity, and guidance, teaching kids to value healthy foods can be an enjoyable adventure.

What is Healthy Eating?

Healthy eating means eating a variety of foods that cover all of the major nutrients like protein, carbohydrates, fats, vitamins, and minerals. Building a nutritious and well-balanced diet that includes all of these nutrients is essential for your child's development as they grow.

It is important for the healthy development of your child. And that's why it is crucial to give children healthy food options that will nourish their bodies and aid brain development. If your child regularly eats a wide variety of basic foods, they would be well-nourished.

How much food is good for your child?

With babies and toddlers, you can usually leave it to them to eat the right amount of food at each meal, as long as you make only healthy foods available.

Babies cry to let us know they're hungry. When they're full, they stop eating. Things get more complicated at age two or three, when children begin to prefer the tastes of certain foods, dislike the tastes of other foods, and have a lot of variation in how hungry they are. But even then it usually works best to make only healthy foods available and let your child decide how much to eat.

It may worry you to see your child eat very little of a meal. Children tend to eat the same number of calories every day if they are allowed to decide how much to eat. But the pattern of calorie intake may vary from day to day. One day a child may eat a big breakfast, a big lunch, and hardly any dinner. The next day this same child may eat very little at breakfast but may eat a lot at lunch and dinner. Don't expect your child to eat the same amount of food at every meal and snack each day. Instead, aim for them to feel satiated and satisfied after each meal.

How can you help your child eat well and be healthy?

Many parents worry that their child is either eating too much or too little. Perhaps your child only wants to eat one type of food; peanut butter and jelly sandwiches, for instance. One way to help your child eat well and help you worry less is to know what your job is and what your child's job is when it comes to eating. If your child only wants to eat one type of food, he or she is doing the parent's job of deciding what food choices are. It is the parent's job to decide what foods are offered.

Your job is to offer nutritious food choices at meals and snack times. You decide the what, where, and when of eating.

Your child's job is to choose how much he or she will eat of the foods you serve. Your child decides how much or even whether to eat.

Giving your children options is important as it lets them have a sense of autonomy. Stock your kitchen and pantry with healthy options and allow them to choose out of this variety. A method often used by parents is the "this or that" method, where children get to pick what they want to eat out of the variety presented by their parents. It encourages some independence and results in better cooperation when it comes to eating.

If this idea is new to you, it may take a little time for both you and your child to adjust. Adhering to your child's every whim when it comes to food can end up creating greater health issues as kids are attracted to sweets and unhealthy foods. However, with time, your child will learn that he or she will be allowed to eat as little or as much as he or she wants at each meal and snack, the key here being that they are fully satiated and have made a choice out of healthy options. This will encourage your child to continue to trust his or her internal hunger gauge.

Here are some ways you can help support your child's healthy eating habits:

Eat together as a family as often as possible. Keep family meals pleasant and positive. Avoid making comments about the amount or type of food your child eats. Pressure to eat actually reduces children's acceptance of new or different foods.

Make healthy food choices for your family's meals. When children notices the choices you make, they will follow your example.

Make meal times fairly consistent and predictable. Fall into a routine of eating at around the same times every day and always at the table, even for snacks.

Have meals often enough (for example, about every three hours for toddlers) so that your child doesn't get too hungry.

Do nothing else during the meal other than talking and enjoying each other—no TV or other distractions.

> Poem Time
>
> *Tick tock goes the clock, and it's 9'oclock in the morning.*
> *What time is nine? It's time to dine on breakfast.*

Fit for a king, hear the timer ping,
We'll gather to munch a tasty, healthy
 breakfast.
The morning is bright, and the kitchen
 shine with sunlight,
As the porridge bubbles on the hob,
the children get excited about the
 wholesome grub.
For breakfast its grains, berries, toast,
 and nuts
With all this variety, breakfast will never
 get stuck in a rut.
A good breakfast packs you with power for
 the day,
And chases worktime worries away.
Slurping up the milk is glorious fun,
Can you see the children smile?
They'll taste the porridge and say to mum,
 "Yum!"
In the spoon goes, sending vitamins to the
 toes,
They'll feel the energy soon,
because from the spoon it goes,
down to their toes.
With a final crunch, they'll be off out the
 door,

> *Until lunchtime comes, and the whole*
> *family will be back at the table once*
> *more!*
> *Tick Tock goes the clock, and it's Eleven*
> *O'clock in the morning.*
> *Listen to the sound of a tummy grumble.*
> *Everyone should stop for a snack at*
> *11'clock in the morning.*
> *Snack time is there to help us work and*
> *play,*
> *for even longer today.*
> *A quick bite to eat will help to keep*
> *strength up and moods at bay.*
> *Tick Tock goes the clock, it ticks all day,*
> *and it ticks all night,*
> *When it chimes for mealtimes, everyone*
> *knows life will be fair.*
> *So, gather to eat at all times of the day,*
> *Sit at the table and say,*
> *"What a wonderful thing food is."*

Here are some other ways you can help your child stay healthy:

Set limit on your child's daily television and computer time.

WHAT IS HEALTHY EATING?

Make physical activity a part of your family's daily life. For example, walk your child to and from school and take a walk after dinner. Teach your young child how to skip, hop, dance, play catch, ride a bike, and more. Encourage your older child to find his or her favorite ways to be active.

Take your child for regular checkups. You can use this time to discuss with a doctor your child's growth rate, activity level, and eating habits.

Poem Time

*The lunch packed, and the lunch box had
    been left open.*
*When all was quiet in the kitchen, and the
    children tucked up to sleep,*
The lunchbox treats jumped to their feet.
*Inside the lunchbox, there was a party
    going on.*
*The string cheese and carrots were singing
    a song.*
*The fruit bar was dancing, and the corn
    was popping.*
*The hummus was ready to splash into
    a dip,*
*And ready for the plunge was the
    wholewheat chip.*

*"I'm the best snack. Look at my bounce,"
sang the chewy fruit bar.*

*"No!" cried the cracker, "I'm the crunchiest,
healthiest snack in town."*

*"Make way for my groove, I swing and
move." said the string cheese as he bent
to his knees.*

*The banana stood tall and ran at the
cheese. "You're not as tall and bendy
as me."*

*"We're rad," said the almonds and walnuts
as they jumped out the bag.*

"Altogether, we go. We can put on a show."

*"Hush, hear that sound!" whispered the
little raisin.*

*"Mum's coming back to pack up the lunch,
the party is over, you healthy bunch."
the banana declared as Mum came
down the stairs and into the kitchen.
She zipped up the lunch box and slid it
into the fridge. If only she knew what
nonsense would go on when the lights
went out.*

What causes poor eating habits?

WHAT IS HEALTHY EATING? | 151

Poor eating habits can develop in otherwise healthy children for several reasons. Infants are born liking sweet tastes. But if babies are going to learn to eat a wide variety of basic foods, they need to learn to enjoy other tastes, because many nutritious foods don't taste sweet.

Ensure that the available food choices are healthy. If candy and soft drinks are always available, most children will gravitate towards these cravings rather than a more nutritious snack. But forbidding these choices can make your child want them even more. You can include some less nutritious foods as part of your child's meals so that he or she learns to enjoy them along with other foods. Try to make a variety of nutritious and appealing food choices available.

Healthy and kid-friendly snack ideas include:

- String cheese.
- Whole wheat crackers and peanut butter.
- Air-popped or low-fat microwave popcorn.
- Frozen juice bars made with 100% real fruit.
- Fruit and dried fruit.
- Baby carrots with hummus or bean dip.
- Low-fat yogurt with fresh fruit.
- The need for personal choice.

Power struggles between a parent and child can affect eating behaviour. If children are pressured to eat a certain food, they are more likely to refuse to eat that food, even if it is something they usually would enjoy. Parents are to provide a variety of nutritious foods and children can decide what and how much they will eat from the choices offered to them.

STORYTIME

Charlotte was a hotheaded four-year-old. She liked the colour pink, drawing with crayons, and most of all, she loved peanut butter sandwiches. Charlotte would refuse to eat anything else. It was a sad, sorry time Charlotte would fold her arms and shake her head.
"I'd rather go straight to bed!" She would say defiantly as a plate of pie and vegetables sat before her. Mum and Dad sighed a deep sigh as the little girl refused another meal of food.
"What will she eat?" Dad asked.
"She'll only eat peanut butter sandwiches."
sighed Mum.
"Peanut butter sandwiches? How silly!" Dad exclaimed. "Eat that pie, Charlotte. I don't want to be here all day."
But Charlotte was a stubborn little child, and her

hair was frizzy and wild. She wouldn't even take a
bite of the smoky steak pie.

"Just one spoonful, go on." Mum pleaded; desperation evident in her voice.

Charlotte slowly looked at the plate, shook her head, and went to find, in the kitchen, some bread, and a butter knife. She went to the cupboard and pulled out a jar of the crunchy, nutty spread.

Mum and Dad were both filled with dread at the sticky jar of peanut butter in the girl's hands.

Charlotte was an expert, you see, in making her very favourite kind of tea. She slapped on the spread and folded the bread, then cut in half and let out a triumphant laugh.

"You'll never feed me anything else except peanut butter sandwiches!" she shouted.

Mum and Dad looked at each other; they were sure that there had to be a severe cure for this little child's obsession with her spread, which came from heaven.

"Straight to bed then, off you go, and don't expect to get any treats when peanut butter is all you eat!" said Dad, although he felt utterly defeated by his stubborn and fussy child.

The little girl went to bed, and Mum and Dad scratched their heads.

"We need to make a plan."

"I know! Let's call Gran."

Gran was a battle-axe of a figure, old and creaky, and she couldn't have been slimmer. But this lady knew a thing or two about fussy little children, and she knew what to do.

"We'll take her to my house, and there she will see that there are many foods that she can have for tea." So, for the first time, Charlotte went to stay with Gran.

Teatime came at the end of the day, and after saying grace, Charlotte looked at the food on her plate.

"You're kidding me, right?" The little girl said. "I only eat peanut butter on bread."

"That's not your choice," Gran said firmly. "Just try this new food, it's delicious."

Charlotte was stunned; she had never been stuck for food before. She wouldn't be able to find any peanut butter in Gran's kitchen drawers.

Charlotte decided to take a bite of the toast. Her taste buds kicked into action as the new flavour floated around her lips, then she swallowed it down.

"It's nice. I love it. It's delicious!" Charlotte gleamed with joy, just as if she was gifted with a new toy.

"So, you like marmite, well, that's a surprise. I've never liked it myself!" said Gran. "Tomorrow, we'll try the damson jam."

> From then on, Charlotte knew that it was often useful to try new foods. After staying with Gran for just one week, Charlotte had a whole range of foods that she would happily eat.
> The End

Emotion. A child's sadness, anxiety, or family crisis can cause undereating or overeating. Food can very quickly become a response to extreme emotions. If you think your child's emotions are affecting his or her eating, focus on resolving the problem that is causing the emotions instead of focusing on the eating behaviour.

If your child is healthy and eating a nutritious and varied diet, yet seems to eat very little, consider that they simply need less food energy (calories) than other children. And some children need more daily calories than others of the same age or size, and they eat more than you might expect. Every child has different calorie needs.

In rare cases, a child may eat more or less than usual because of a medical condition that affects his or her appetite. If your child has a medical condition that affects how he or she eats, talk with your child's doctor about how you can help your child get the right amount of nutrition.

What are the risks of eating poorly?

A child with poor eating habits is going to be poorly nourished. That means they won't be getting the amounts of nutrients needed to foster healthy growth and development. This can lead to being underweight or overweight. Poorly nourished children tend to have weaker immune systems, which increases their chances of illness. Poor eating habits can increase a child's risk for heart disease, high blood pressure, type 2 diabetes, or high cholesterol later in life.

Poor eating habits include:

- Eating a very limited variety of foods.
- Eating too many foods of poor nutritional quality, such as soft drinks, chips, and doughnuts.
- Overeating from being served large portions or being told to "clean your plate" or "finish it all up."

Make Small Changes

You should make healthy food choices for your family's meals. Children will usually notice the choices you make and follow your example. Start with small, easy-to-achieve changes, such as offering more fruits and vegetables at meals and snacks.

Set up a regular snack and meal schedule. Most children do well with three meals and two or three snacks a day.

Find at least one food from each food group that your child likes. Make sure it is readily available most of the time.

Serve breakfast. Having breakfast with your child can help start a lifelong healthy habit.

Let your child drink no more than one small cup of juice per day. Encourage your child to rely on water to quench their thirst, rather than sweet, sugary drinks.

Avoid buying junk food. Get healthy snacks that your child likes, and keep them within easy reach. Healthy and kid-friendly snacks.

Ideas include:

- String cheese.

- Whole wheat crackers and peanut butter.

- Fruit and dried fruit.

- Baby carrots with hummus or bean dip.

- Low-fat yoghurt with fresh fruit.

Healthy eating doesn't mean that your child has to give up all of their favourite treats. Those types of foods are acceptable when consumed in moderation now and then. The key is to strike a balance between all of these different types of foods and guide your child to a well-balanced diet.

Share the Responsibility

You decide when, where, and what the family eats. Your child chooses whether and how much to eat from the options you provide. Young children are good at listening to their bodies. They eat when they're hungry and stop when they're full. When you try to control how much children eat, you interfere with this natural ability. Understand that as your child grows, relinquishing some control is required from the parent for your children to accept these new changes and mature accordingly. Keeping this division of responsibility helps your child stay in touch with those internal cues.

Help your children learn to eat slowly and recognize when they are full. Don't let rules, pleading, or bargaining dictate your child's eating patterns.

Physical Activity

One of the best things you can do for your child's health is to help make physical activity a habit. If physical activity is a habit for you, it will more likely become a habit for your children.

Find ways for your child to be active for at least 1-hour each day. Children can break up the time into several 10- to 15-minute periods of vigorous exercise throughout the day.

STORYTIME

After a rainy weekend, the sun finally came out on the first Monday of the school holidays.

Johnny had been playing video games all weekend. When he woke up, he went to play on the Xbox. After lunch, Johnny played a car racing game, and before bed, he played on Minecraft.

"I love Xbox so much that I'll never do anything else," he told his friend Max.

Just as Johnny was in the middle of completing the very highest level, the TV screen fizzled and fluttered with grey lines. The colours went all fuzzy, and suddenly, the video game crashed, and the whole TV screen turned black.

"What's going on with my Xbox?!" he shouted at the top of his voice. He pressed the button again and again, but the machine would not restart.

"What on earth should I do now that my TV is broken?" he wondered.

"Let's go and play outside. The sun is shining," said Max.

"Oh, alright, but I don't want to do any exercise," Johnny mumbled.

"Don't be silly," said Max. "Exercise is super fun."

The boys ran down to the park, and Max brought a ball and his badminton rackets. At first, Johnny didn't want to play and wasn't sure of himself, but soon, he was just as enthusiastic as Max in kicking the ball. It wasn't long before Max and Johnny had so much fun that Johnny had almost forgotten his broken TV.

"My legs feel full of energy, and my heart is beating fast!" said Johnny as he chased the ball around the park.

"That's why I like to go out to play every day!" said Max, "Do you want to come to the swimming pool with my family tomorrow?"

Johnny scratched his head and wondered. He had never been to a swimming pool before. He remembered dipping his toes in the sea on holiday once, and it was freezing.

"I don't know, swimming isn't for me." he shook his head.

"Come on, and it will be fun, give it a try!" Max persuaded.

Johnny thought that since his TV was damaged, he wouldn't be able to play video games tomorrow, and maybe it would be a good idea to spend some time with Max's family. So, the next day, Johnny was excited to splash in the pool. He jumped in full speed and laughed loudly.

"What a splash!" Max's dad commented.

"So, when do you think you'll be able to fix your Xbox?" said Max as they came out of the swimming pool.

Johnny replied, "Oh yeah! I completely forgot about my Xbox, to be honest. I've had so much fun outdoors, and I don't think I'll need to get it fixed for at least another week!"

Johnny was looking forward to the next week, even without his Xbox. He was excited about the activities he had planned with Max.

The End

Make it Fun

Don't force your children to exercise. Labelling it as "exercise" simply turns it into another chore that they must do. Exercise comes in plenty of forms, and the options are endless to find activities that your children will enjoy. Simply make physical activity part of daily routines.

• Jump rope, dance, skate, or play Frisbee with your child.

• Walk with your child to do errands, or walk to the bus stop or school, if possible.

• Have your child invite a friend over once a week for an activity, such as a bike ride, a water balloon fight, or building a snow fort.

- Let your child try different organized activities to see what he or she enjoys, such as tennis, T-ball, soccer, or martial arts.

- Let your child pick out a low-cost toy that promotes activity, such as a jump rope, Frisbee, or ball.

- Frequently, leaving your children to their own devices with their friends leads to active play. Allow them to get bored because it encourages them to come up with their games and ways to entertain themselves.

Get the whole Family Involved

When the whole family is involved in physical activities together, children learn that being active is fun and makes you feel good.

- Ride bikes, walk, fly a kite, or hike together.

- Give family members tasks such as sweeping, weeding, or washing the car.

- Take your family to the park or pool.

- Join other families for group activities like touch football, basketball, or hide-and-seek.

Healthy Habits, Happy Child

What are the healthy habits your child needs to be a happy child. We are talking about healthy emotional habits a happy child needs. The emotional needs of your child are very important.

As a parent, your first responsibility is to support and promote the emotional, intellectual, as well as the physical wellbeing of your child. Unfortunately, most parents are often unsure of how to go about this for fear of making mistakes. But know that most things with parenting require trial and error. Some children may respond well with specific strategies, while others may not have such a positive result. Parenting classes are not widely taught. So the first thing that is needed is educated parents. Without educating yourself, you will have a hard time helping your child develop into a normal emotionally healthy member of society.

Parenting has taken some hits in recent years because we seem to have gotten away from the basics. In most cases parents are not completely at fault. Times have really changed and our family dynamics have changed with it. Today parenting management guides are readily available that deal with today's new challenges.

The goal here is to give the parent or caregiver some very basic healthy emotional habits to allow you to raise a happy child. Below are six basic healthy habits you should try and implement into your everyday life. Make notes on each one on how you can implement these healthy habits into your daily routine.

Emotional Security

You should help protect your child's psyche by providing a safe loving environment. Provide an environment with a sense of being loved, needed, and welcomed. Throw in a little encouragement regularly.

Emotional Development

Always remember to lead by example. Show your capacity for compassion, and empathy towards the sick, weaker, and older. If you still have grandparents available, include them in your children's activity whenever possible to show them the diversity and range of people that they will encounter in their lives. New social situations expose them to new emotions, some more uncomfortable than the last. But by doing so, you can give your children the blueprint on what to do in certain situations so that they understand how to channel their emotions and convey them appropriately.

Physical Security

Physical security is exactly what it means, the safety of a child's body and life. Also, it is providing food, shelter, clothes etc. Show your child you care about their security by warning them of dangers in their world and the bigger world. There are so many dangers now with the Internet and as children become more accustomed to the online world, educating them on the dangerous side of something that may seem innocent at first is incredibly important. Prepare your children, in addition to monitoring them, especially when they are young.

Physical Development

As children age, they develop physical changes that will differ from their parents, their mentors, and other children. Provide the opportunity for appropriate conditions for physical exercise. Children need physical activity to develop normally. They also need the right education to prepare them for the changes their body will be experiencing. Plan and be open to talking to children about the new things they are experiencing, especially with their bodies. Physical development should never be a shameful thing and treat it as such when guiding your children.

Intellectual Security

It is important that your child's mind can develop without prejudices. Develop a habit of listening openly to your child's ideas. Guide their thoughts with respect and dignity. Don't be afraid to correct with facts but be mindful of their beliefs and foster a safe space where they can share their feelings, thoughts and opinions. The last thing you want is for your child to be afraid to share their ideas or be closed off from you. Even if there are differences between your thoughts, be open to understanding their point of view and remember that everyone's opinions can change, yours included.

Intellectual Development

Supply a safe and secure environment for learning. This will include all the mistakes the learning process requires. Discuss the learning mistakes your child makes openly and fairly, always encouraging them to keep learning.

A child's work is called play. A child's play will include all three areas of development: emotional, physical, and intellectual development. Parenting healthy habits allows your child to participate in all three areas equally.

If you can get into these healthy habits with your child you will soon have a happy child that develops naturally. Remember, these healthy habits will be ongoing and implemented throughout your child's life.

HEALTHY DRINKS FOR KIDS

Although it can be challenging to get your child to eat healthier foods, it can be just as challenging to find safe and enticing drinks for your kids.

Most kids have a sweet tooth and are likely to request sugar. But it is vital for their overall health to direct them towards safer options.

Below are some recommended drinks for kids — as well as three drinks to avoid.

Water

You should always give water first when your child tells you they are thirsty.

This fact is necessary because water is vital for your child's health and essential for countless critical processes, including temperature control and organ functioning. Kids are intelligent and understand simple concepts like this. Explaining why water is so crucial and why sodas have the opposite effect can illustrate to children why their parents are so adamant on water, thus leading them to have a deeper understanding. While they may not always agree with you and may insist on wanting a sugary drink, knowing that your child understands its importance already puts them miles ahead.

Kids have higher water requirements than adults due to their rapidly growing body and higher metabolic rate. Unlike many other foods, water does not contain liquid calories, making your child less likely to feel full and resist solid food. This formula is useful if your child has a small appetite.

Also, drinking ample water has to do with healthy body weight, decreased risk of dental cavities, and enhanced brain development in kids.

Furthermore, dehydration may have a detrimental effect on your child's health in several ways, potentially reducing brain activity, causing constipation and fatigue.

Get your kids used to drinking, reaching for water instead of sweet, flavoured drinks.

Naturally Flavored Water

Since plain water may seem dull, this vital fluid will not be loved by your infant.

Try to infuse the water with fresh fruits and herbs to make it more exciting without adding additional sugar and calories.

To find out what your child loves, you can try several flavour variations.

Also, your child is strengthened by the fresh fruit and herbs used in the water.

Such winning combinations include:

- Pineapple and mint
- Blueberries and raspberries
- Strawberries and lemon
- Cucumber and watermelon
- Orange and lime

Engage your child to select their desired flavour combination and help add ingredients to the drink. Getting your kids involved in this process encourages them to want to drink the final product.

Stores also sell reusable water bottles with integrated infusers that are relatively inexpensive. These are a great way to help your child stay hydrated, especially when away from home and not under your supervision.

Coconut Water

While the coconut water contains calories and sugar, the option is healthier than other beverages such as soda and sports drinks. Coconut water has the right quantity of nutrients – all of which are essential, including vitamin C, magnesium, and potassium.

It also includes electrolytes — such as potassium, magnesium, calcium, and sodium — that are lost during exercise by sweat.

This fact makes coconut water an outstanding moisture alternative to healthy kids' sports drinks.

Coconut water is also helpful when your child is sick, especially if they need rehydration after diarrhoea or vomiting.

However, when buying coconut water, it is necessary to read the label carefully. Be wary of some brands that add extra sugars and artificial flavours. The best choice for kids is pure, unsweetened coconut water, always.

Certain Smoothies

Smoothies are a scrupulous way to move your child's diet into fruits, vegetables, and other nutritious foods. Not only do they taste delicious, but an exciting new concoction for your children to dabble into.

While some premade smoothies are filled with sugar, homemade smoothies make excellent choices for kids, as long as they're rich in nutritious ingredients.

Parents coping with picky eaters find smoothies incredibly helpful. Many vegetables — such as kale, spinach, and even cauliflower — can be combined into a tasty smoothie your kid would love.

Such child-friendly variations of smoothie include:

- Kale and pineapple
- Strawberries and beets
- Peach and cauliflower
- Spinach and blueberries

Combine non-dairy milk or soy products and use organic add-ins, such as hemp seeds, cacao powder, unsweetened chocolate, avocado, or ground flax seeds.

Avoid buying smoothies at supermarkets or restaurants, since they can contain added sugars and prefer homemade versions whenever possible. Since smoothies are high in calories, make them a snack or a small meal.

Consider freezing your smoothies in ice cream moulds. These are a fantastic and healthy treat that excite your kids, especially since they are served on a stick, like ice cream.

Unsweetened Milk

While many kids prefer sweetened milk drinks such as chocolate or strawberry milk, the kids' healthier alternative is straightforward, unsweetened milk.

Simple milk is highly nutritious and supplies many nutrients necessary for growth and development.

Milk contains protein, calcium, phosphorus, and magnesium, such as vital nutrients for bone health, particularly for kids growing up.

Also, vitamin D is another essential bone vitamin, which is fortified. Although many parents prefer to give kids fat-free milk, milk with higher fat content is better for younger kids because fat is essential for proper brain development and overall development.

Because of an increased metabolic rate, kids have a higher need for fat than adults.

This fact is the reason for higher fat milk options, such as 2% fat milk, which are healthier for most kids than skimmed milk.

However, you should also keep in mind that consuming too much milk can lead kids to get full and potentially eat less of their meals or snacks. To ensure your child is not loaded with milk before consuming food, give only a small amount of milk at mealtime.

While milk is a nutritious drink, many kids are intolerant of milk. Milk sensitivity is characterized by bloating, diarrhoea, vomiting, skin rashes, and abdominal cramps.

Talk to your doctor if you are allergic to milk.

Unsweetened Plant-Based Milk

Unsweetened plant milk is an ideal choice for kids who are intolerant to raw milk. There are several alternatives when it comes to dairy-free milk, and many of them taste delicious and avoid the stomach sensitivities that may come with regular milk.

Milk on plants contains cotton, chocolate, almond, cassava, rice, and soymilk.

Sweetened milk can contain much-added sugar and artificial sweeteners, including sweetened milk, so it is best to use unsweetened varieties.

Use unsweetened herbal milk as a low-calorie drink on its own or a foundation for child-friendly smoothies, oatmeals, and soups. For example, 1 cup of unsweetened almond milk (240 ml) has less than 40 calories.

Providing low-calorie drinks with food reduces your child's risk of filling liquids alone. Many vegetable milks contain a range of vitamins and minerals and are often enhanced by nutrients such as calcium, B12, and vitamin D.

Certain Herbal Teas

While tea is not commonly considered a child-friendly drink, some herbal teas are safe and healthy for kids.

Herbal teas — such as orange, mint, rooibos, and camomile — are excellent choices for sweetened drinks as they are free of caffeine and have a good taste.

Herbal teas can provide health benefits and can also support sick or nervous kids.

For starters, camomile and lemongrass teas have been used for a long time to soothe anxiety in both kids and adults alike.

Use Camomile for both kids and adults as a natural cure for digestive symptoms, including nausea, vomiting, diarrhoea, and indigestion.

Research shows that camomile has anti-inflammatory effects and can help alleviate intestinal inflammatory symptoms.

Although some herbal teas are considered safe for kids, before giving your child any herbal teas, it is necessary to check with your paediatrician.

Bear in mind as well that herbal teas are not ideal for babies and should be consumed healthily to avoid burning infants.

Drinks to Limit

Although it is entirely appropriate for kids to enjoy a sweetened drink occasionally; you should not give them access to sugary drinks daily.

Frequent consumption of sweetened drinks — such as soda and sports drinks — can contribute to health conditions such as obesity and dental cavities in kids.

Many of these drinks also contain additives that are addictive for children, so getting them to stop their reliance on these drinks will pose as a huge challenge.

Soda and Sweetened Beverages

Soda, and other sweetened beverages such as sports drinks, sweetened milk, and sweet teas, that should be limited in a child's diet.

A standard Coca-Cola's 12-ounce (354-ml) serving includes 39 grams of sugar — or almost ten teaspoons.

The American Heart Organization (AHO) recommends that kids aged 2–18 keep less than six teaspoons (25 grams) per day. Sweetened drinks are connected with increased risk of disease in kids, such as type 2 diabetes and non-alcoholic fatty liver disease.

Furthermore, drinking too many sweetened drinks can lead to kids' weight gain and cavities.

Moreover, many sweetened beverages, including condensed milk, contain fructose-high corn syrup, a refined sweetener associated with kids' weight gain.

Juice

Although 100 % fruit juice supplies essential vitamins and minerals, you should limit them to the quantities prescribed for kids. Medical organizations, such as the US Academy of Pediatrics (AAP), suggest that for kids between 1-6 years and 8-12 ounces (236-355 ml) per day, the juice is limited to 4-6 ounces (120-180 ml) per day.

Usually, 100% fruit juice is not related to weight gain when consumed in these quantities.

Excessive intake of fruit juice in kids is, however, associated with an increased risk of obesity.

Also, some studies have related the daily consumption of fruit juice to weight gain for younger kids.

An analysis of 8 studies revealed, for example, kids aged 1–6 who consumed 100% fruit juice have an increased gain in weight over one year.

As the filling fiber in whole fresh fruit is absent from fruit juice, it is easy for kids to drink consume too much, thus exceeding the acceptable sugar consumption amounts as prescribed by experts.

For these purposes, kids can, wherever possible, consume whole fruit instead of fruit juice.

The AAP recommends that the juice of infants under one year of age be fully limited.

Caffeinated Beverages

Many young kids consume caffeine drinks — such as soda, coffee, and power drinks — that can adversely affect health. One study found that about 75% of U.S. kids aged 6–19 use caffeine, with an average consumption of 25 mg per day of 2–11-year-olds and twice as high for kids between 12 and 17.

Caffeine can lead to jitteriness, fast heart rate, high blood pressure, anxiety, and kids' sleep disturbances, which is why age-based caffeinated drinks should be limited. Caffeine should be limited to not more than 85–100 mg a day for kids older than 12 in kids' health organizations like the AAP and should be avoided in kids under 12.

Parents should bear in mind that some energy drinks can contain more than 100 mg of caffeine per 12-ounce serving (354 ml) to prevent excessive coffee consumption.

Bonus Tip: Easy and Healthy Smoothies for Kids

A smoothie consists of raw vegetable, fruit, dairy products, mixed juice such as milk or yoghurt. It can also be 100% fruit or vegetables or both, without dairy products. The creamy texture can attract kids to a smoothie. You can also combine fruit with vegetables and to get the most nutrients out of a glass.

Smoothies can be safe during breakfast or evening snacks. They can be easily made for those who are on-the-go and are suitable for busy parents and kids. But if your child likes to eat fruit, it's nice to give it in its entirety because eating the fruit allows for it to break down slowly in our digestive systems to absorb the healthy compounds and thus prevent a sugar spike.

We will share some exciting smoothies for kids in this chapter.

The awareness of smoothies has encouraged businesses to come up with ready-to-go smoothies in different flavours.

Although it's all right to have a packed smoothie, sometimes, homemade smoothies made from fresh fruits and vegetables are much better.

Make sure you read the labels thoroughly to know the ingredients when purchasing a ready-to-use smoothie. Select low sodium smoothies with no added sugar.

Green Smoothies for Kids

These smoothies are made from dark green vegetables and leafy vegetables and filled with essential nutrients. All of these recipes can be whipped up within 10 minutes, including prep time for all of the fruits and vegetables. While these recipes are tried and tested, smoothies are a great way to use up veggies and fruits in your refrigerator. Some of the best smoothies are made without a recipe! These are a great guideline, but smoothies are also perfect for experimentation and finding your favourite combination. You can never really go wrong with smoothies!

Kale Banana Smoothie

This smoothie is a seamless mixture of ingredients that create a delicious and healthy blend of vitamins and minerals. Kale and banana are filled with healthy fats from flaxseed and soymilk.

Ingredients

- Two cups of chopped kale
- One pair of ripe bananas
- One tsp of flax seeds
- ½ cup unsweetened soy milk
- One tsp of maple syrup

Preparation:

- Blend the flax seeds
- Mix the banana, chopped kale, maple syrup, and soy milk to the blender and blend for two mins.
- Serve fresh.

Apple Smoothie Spinach

Do your kids dislike spinach? Mix its flavour with apple and banana in this recipe. The smoothie also includes yoghurt, which is a probiotic source. It also contains prebiotic ingredients. This recipe is an excellent pre-probiotic blend mixture to give your kid a healthy gut.

Ingredients

- One cup chopped spinach leaves
- One ripe banana

- 1/2 apple, peeled and chopped
- One cup of grapes, preferably seedless
- One tub of vanilla cream yoghurt

Preparation:

- Cut the banana (peel excluded) and put away the seeds of the grape.
- Put the banana, chopped spinach leaves, grapes, yoghurt, and apple in a blender and blend for two mins, or until you achieve a smooth mixture.
- Serve fresh.

Honeydew Melon Cucumber Smoothie

This smoothie is good to try in summer because the ingredients produce a calm feeling that is very important. This recipe also helps to improve the rehydration of multivitamins and multi-minerals.

Ingredients

- One honeydew melon
- One cup of green grapes, preferably seedless
- One cucumber peeled and diced
- 1/4 cup mint leaves

Preparation

- Peel, cut seeds, and dice the honeydew melon.
- Add melon cubes, green grapes, cucumber, and mint leaves and blend for a minute. Blend together.
- Serve cool.

Spinach and Kale Smoothie

If your kids refuse to eat dark green vegetables or leafy ones, encourage them to drink them. Spinach and Kale is a recipe for a healthy yet tasty green smoothie for kids.

Ingredients

- Two cups of chopped spinach leaves
- One tbsp of peanut butter
- One kale leaf
- One sliced of banana, frozen or fresh
- One cup of almond milk

Preparation

- Clean and cut the spinach and kale leaves.
- Add the spinach, kale, and almond milk to a blender and puree for a minute or until you've got a smooth mix.

- Add the banana and blend for another 30 seconds or until the perfect consistency is reached.
- Serve cool.

Papaya Smoothie

Papayas and potassium, calcium, and magnesium minerals are abundant in A, and C. Fiber and antioxidants are in the fruit to help your kids stay healthy.

Ingredients

- One papaya, peeled and diced
- One cup of low-fat yoghurt
- 1/2 cup pineapple chunks
- One tsp of coconut extract
- One tsp of flaxseed
- Crushed ice

Preparation

- Cut and dice the papaya.
- In the mixer, add pieces of papaya, pineapple chunks, yoghurt, coconut extract, linseed, and ice and blend for one minute or until a mixture is smooth.

- Apply consistency water and mix again for a couple of seconds.
- Serve.

Creamy Date Smoothie

Dates are sweet, low in sodium, and high in fiber. They have minerals like potassium, magnesium, zinc, A, K, riboflavin, folate, thiamine, and niacin.

Ingredients

- 1/3 cup of halved or pitted dates
- 3/4 of cup milk
- 1/2 of cup crushed ice

Preparation

- Mix the dates with milk for one minute.
- Remove the ice crushed and blend for another 30 seconds.
- Serve cool.

Berry Smoothie

This smoothie is a healthy breakfast choice for your child with antioxidants.

Ingredients

- One cup of fresh or frozen berries – strawberries, raspberries, blueberries
- One cup of low-fat yoghurt
- Two small bananas
- 1/2 cup of crushed ice

Preparation

- Blend the berries, yoghurt, sliced bananas, and ice for a minute or until the necessary consistency is achieved.
- Serve cool.

Green Grape Smoothie

The grapes contain ample vitamin C and antioxidants. Their sweet and delicate tastes make the green smoothie delicious. Here's how to make a grape smoothie for kids.

Ingredients

- Two cups of grapes, preferably seedless
- One banana, frozen or fresh
- A handful of Italian parsley
- One cup of spinach leaves

- 1/2 cup of low-fat milk or water

Preparation

- Wash well the spinach and grapes.
- Slice the banana and, if any, separate the grapes from the seeds.
- Mix all ingredients and drink.

Banana Smoothie

Potassium and vitamin C are high in this smoothie; it is one of the easiest fruit smoothies you can make for your kids. Cinnamon powder is a source of antioxidants and other bioactive anti-inflammatory compounds. The ingredient mix in this recipe will improve your infant's health.

Ingredients

- Two bananas
- One cup of milk, preferably low-fat
- Two tablespoons of brown sugar
- Water for consistency
- Ice cubes (optional)
- Cinnamon powder (optional)

Preparation

- Mix the banana and milk until the fruit is cut or sliced.
- Apply brown sugar and water and blend for 10 seconds again.
- Add ice if you like, blend the mixture for a minute again.
- Top it with ground cinnamon and serve chilled.
- If you want a milk-free smoothie, you may supplement standard milk with soy milk or almond milk.

Blueberry Smoothie

Here's a delicious blueberry smoothie recipe for your kids.

Ingredients

- One cup of blueberries – fresh or frozen
- One cup of plain yoghurt
- ½ cup of soy milk
- Two tbsp of white sugar
- A pinch of nutmeg powder
- ½ tsp of vanilla extract

Preparation

- Wash blueberries for a minute with yoghurt and add milk to make a smooth combination.
- Add nutmeg powder, sugar, and water and combine until you have a perfect consistency.
- Serve cool.

You should give your kids a wide variety of nutritious beverages always.

Infused plain water, milk, herbal milk, and certain herbal teas are examples of kid-friendly drinks.

Instead of sugar and high-calorie beverages, such as soda, milk, and sports drinks, you can use these drinks.

While your child may object to exchanging their favourite sweetened drink for a healthier alternative, be sure you're doing the right thing for your child's health.

HEALTHY NUTRITION FOR KIDS

As we know, nutrition is critical for a child's learning process and development. Some might even argue that nutrition is the key to raising a healthy, happy child. This itself holds some weight to it, as health plays such a huge factor in our emotions and moods, which affects everything we do. Establishing the right habits as a child decides how healthy they will be when he or she becomes an adult. Even though experts unanimously agree that kids should get their nutritional requirements from a healthy and balanced diet, unfortunately, many children do not eat such a diet regularly, leading to deficiency-related medical issues. In such cases, nutritional supplements give the missing ingredients of the diet.

Having healthy kids is something that we all want. Raising healthy children will depend on the balance of a number of things since children have to be healthy in all aspects. Generally, children who are healthy are thriving and will perform better in everything that they do.

Mentally, you can help stimulate your child's development by teaching them the different skills that they need. Reading stories together daily, talking about the things that they did, and helping your child find out what their interests are will all help. Allow your child to explore the world around them so that they learn about how things work and they are able to satisfy their curiosity. Engage in conversation with your child and take things in from their perspective. The world is a big place, and for them, grappling with all of these new faces, sounds and sensations can be incredibly overwhelming. This is where parents step in as a constant pillar of support.

In terms of emotions, a lot of support should be given in their areas of interest. Take time to praise your child for the good things that they do and try to keep away from negative remarks. Instead, provide commentary that is honest and realistic as well as constructive.

Every child experiences stress so teach them how to relax and cope with the daily stress that they go through. Listening to what your child has to say is an important part of it all as well, so do make sure to lend an ear and always make eye contact to make them feel that they are important and that their opinion counts too.

Socially, you can help your child develop by exposing them to peers and helping them learn to socialize. Trips to the park, play school and even play dates can help open doors to meeting peers. This can also be a perfect chance for you to teach your child social graces, during situations that call for it.

In the physical aspect, you can raise healthy kids by keeping them active. This does not only mean keeping them playing sports, but also making sure that you both do activities together. Playing with your child can be exercise in itself, and it will help you bond together as well. Of course, you will also need to make sure that your child has the right nutrition in order to grow properly physically.

A well-balanced diet that is properly planned will help ensure that your kids receive the proper nutrition to grow and have the right amount of energy to keep up with daily activities. Good nutrition should be practiced right from the start if you want to raise healthy kids. From the time that you have your child you should make the choice to go natural, picking breast milk over formula. Incorporate as many fruits and vegetables in meals as you can and opt for water or fresh fruit juices when it comes to drinks. If you start early then it will be easier to continue this practice as your child grows older.

A good rule of thumb to follow when trying to raise healthy kids and plan nutritious meals is to stay away from processed foods that can contain additives, chemicals and preservatives. Rather opt for natural and fresh foods that will be better for your kids. Both malnutrition and obesity can be avoided if you keep meals healthy and natural. Keeping this in mind, make it a habit to read the nutritional labels on the things that you buy; you will basically want less of the fats and more of the nutrients such as vitamins and fiber etc.

You can also make sure that your child gets the right nutrition by monitoring what they eat. Instead of having them buy food in the cafeteria where they can get junk from vending machines, try brown bagging. This does not have to mean that meals will be bland and taste awful. It can be a good challenge for you to come up with an interesting and delicious meal that will make your child look forward to lunch each day. Parents also enjoy involving their kids in planning meals. Get your kids in the kitchen; it should never be a space for just the parents. With the right supervision, you can teach your kids basic ways to make their own lunches that they will be more motivated to eat.

As a whole, raising healthy kids is possible if you remember to strike a good balance in all the aspects and give your kids the food they need.

Who Needs Dietary Supplements?

Normally growing children do not necessarily need extra nutritional supplements. Although many young children are picky eaters, it does not necessarily mean that they have nutritional deficiencies. Regular meals and snacks give all the vitamins and minerals that growing children need. Doctors recommend supplements for fussy eaters who do not eat regular and well-balanced meals cooked from whole, fresh foods. Kids who have certain medical conditions such as respiratory and digestive problems may need to supplement their diet. Very active kids who play physically demanding games and sports would be better off by supplementation. Strict vegetarians may need an iron supplement, while a dairy-free diet that is deficient in calcium will need this mineral supplementation. Children who consume fast and processed foods, as well as carbonated drinks that leach out vitamins and minerals from the body, need supplementation with the required nutrients.

Dietary Supplementation to Prevent Childhood Deficiencies

The idealistic approach to kids nutrition of a well-balanced and nutritious diet may not always be realistic. Hence, childhood deficiencies may occur, which could be overcome with the help of nutritional supplements. Supplementing the diet with cod liver oil is necessary to give adequate amounts of omega-3 fatty acids for good brain development in children. As a result of a healthy digestive system, probiotics play a vital role in our bodies by preventing the growth of harmful organisms in the digestive tract. This indirectly translates into good overall health. Although not required in very large-good quality multivitamins and trace minerals quantities, are necessary for the general physical wellbeing. Some studies have stressed the importance of adequate amounts of vitamin K in the body for proper blood clotting. Insufficient amounts of vitamin D in the body may negatively affect many body systems ranging from the brain and immune health to cardiovascular and musculoskeletal health.

Safe Dietary Supplementation for Children

The safety and effectiveness of many of the herbal medicines and dietary supplements may still not have been tested on children, making it all the more imperative that these products be used only under medical supervision. This is because some supplements may interfere with medications that the child is already taking. Even though multivitamins are not recommended for children who eat a balanced diet, doctors recommend this for fussy eaters who do not consume a varied diet. However, a large dose of vitamins or megavitamins is not recommended for kids. Excessive amounts of fat-soluble vitamins, A, D, E, and K may prove toxic for kids.

Health and wellness in the 21st century have some significant problems. We're told we have an obesity epidemic, especially among children, but it is not an obesity problem. It is a health problem. The kids and health challenges can be solved.

Let us look at the big picture. Two variables pop up, both of which need to be addressed to resolve the health problem with kids and adults. We need to make a commitment and take action along these two fronts. When we talk about our children's health, we want to prepare them for healthy adulthood. We want them to live long lives without the debilitating diseases that adults currently face.

We must take action in these two areas:

- Nutrition
- Environment

For kids to be healthy, they need to learn to eat healthy food. We must minimize, if not eliminate, processed foods, foods grown on nutrient-depleted soils, and foods that have to travel around the world before they find their way to our tables.

We need to go local, go organic, and shop at farmer's markets to keep our children from becoming junk food junkies.

If you think organic is too expensive, you can buy wholesale from nearby organic farms by forming co-ops with your friends and neighbours. It will pay dividends in yours and your kids' health. Nutrition once only came from food, but now we also turn to multivitamins that can help us where food falls short.

Kids nutrition should be looked at from when they are newborns to the time they stop growing and become adults. Those needs are different, so we need to speak to those differences. Kids are growing. We want to make sure that they have the kind of nutrition to make strong healthy bones, healthy hearts, and good immune systems. Infants, for example, have weak immune systems which is why mothers' milk helps them get started until they develop their immune systems

We can get multivitamin & multi-mineral powder for infants, a chewable multivitamin for growing kids and teens love meal shakes, fast food with no guilt.

With growing percentages of children visiting medical practitioners to be treated for diseases, illnesses and allergies related to food, we need to address some basic root causes. With their minds and bodies being so young, it is the optimum time to begin teaching them the important lessons for their life on how to truly take care of themselves, and health is the priority. After all, what they learn IS what they know. The following are some easy steps to integrate into your kids's daily routine to begin ingraining healthy habits into their lives.

1. To begin, let's start with water. Every morning and throughout the day, introduce a new simple habit:

Start with water. The average adult's body consists of up to 70% water. It is necessary to survive. It is necessary in every function of our body. Some of these functions include regulating the temperature of the body, humidifying the air we breathe, and it helps organs assimilate the nutrients and expel the toxins and excess salts. It is a mainstay in optimum health of all of our cells, so we need water.

And most of us do not replace the amount lost on a daily basis because we have not created the habit to do so. Instead, we reach for a sugary drink! First thing in the morning when you wake up your children after family devotions should be to go to the kitchen, get into the habit of having at least one full glass of water. Throughout the day, have a glass prior to each meal and snack and then 1 or 2 before bedtime.

The easy association is, if you are going to be putting something into your mouth, ensure you start with water. Try to work yourself up to the amount of 8 glasses each day. This extra water will fill you up, and decrease the amount of food you feel like you need, and may prevent excess unhealthy snacking.

2. Ensure fresh fruits and vegetables are always convenient and accessible to your children when it is time for a snack or meal.

Make sure they learn that each time they eat, something from this valuable food group is to be included. They also need to be taught to wash off all fruits and vegetables prior to eating and learn about the poisons used on many crops we are exposed to in the markets. Teach them the value in buying organic, as our bodies do not get as much exposure to toxins which hinder and cripple our body systems and functions.

3. Plan meals together and get them to help with preparation by having a list of tasks that need to be done at each meal time and have them rotate the tasks.

For example: table setting and cleaning, and meal choice and preparation. Have them plan a list of healthy meals for the week. If their meal is the one chosen for the night, have them help you prepare it and explain the process as you go and the nutritional content of each ingredient. Have them dish out the meal onto the plates with the correct portions for each food type.

Teach them about cleanliness while preparing meals. And most importantly, ensure you praise them throughout. One of the greatest rewards with preparing a meal, is the enjoyment the nourishment can bring to others, their enjoyment of the flavours, as well as the appreciation for the effort it took to create it. Make this part of dinnertime fun! Play music, laugh or smile to let your children know that having fun in the kitchen preparing healthy meals doesn't have to be boring like they might think it to be.

4. After they have chosen meals for the week, get them to create a grocery list to accommodate their menus and take them grocery shopping.

Teach them about the nutritional content in the items they are needing by comparing them to other items with less nutritional value in the store (eg: fresh products used to make meals from scratch as opposed to canned products). Show them how to read food labels and the dangerous ingredients to avoid, like excess sugars or certain kinds of fats.

Teach them the necessity of choosing organic, whole foods without additives, preservatives, genetically modified and hormone enhanced. Smaller delis and markets can offer more specialised healthier products, and their owners will be more than happy to help in the teaching process.

This helps with picky eaters in particular. By giving them a choice and the autonomy to make their own decisions, it helps them feel more motivated to eat. Always consider getting your kids involved, whether it is at the grocery store or in the kitchen.

5. Understand that fear of new foods is practically universal among children. Encourage your child to try out small amounts of new foods at the beginning of a meal when he/she is hungry.

Children have more taste buds than adults and the flavours in foods are heightened so be aware of this and appreciate it. There is a reason liver and onions is on the seniors menu selection and not the children's section. It becomes an acQuired taste as we lose our sensitivities to the harsh flavour of the liver. Offer the child small samples of new foods that adults are enjoying to stimulate the child's natural curiosity. Never force or bribe your child to try a new food, as it almost always erases any preference the child would have developed for the food otherwise. If they don't like the flavor today, this is okay. Appreciate their uniQue pallet but at the same time, realise they are developing a new pallet for new flavors on their own. You should try again at a later date. It is recommended to try in a month. And try the item in a different manner, for example they didn't like tomatoes in a salad, chop them up and put them in a sandwich with other flavours to mask it slightly. Work them into this new flavour. The key here is to provide your children with opportunities to enhance their pallet, never to force them to eat something they don't seem interested in.

6. Use items other than food to reward good behaviour more often than not.

Make a trip to the park or library rather than out for icecream. When kids associate rewards with junk and unhealthy foods, it becomes all the more desirable to them. Eventually, this desire for bad food becomes a habit. On the other hand, banning a child from eating a favourite food makes them yearn for it more, too. So keep minimal amounts of "junk" food, (maybe those special chocolates for special occasions or special days), in an adult only place to be doled out as seen fit by the parent. They will come to learn each time they receive them, that they are in fact a special occasional treat with little to no nutritional content, which is why they don't receive them on a regular basis.

Everyone wants their kids to be healthy. We want them to grow up fast, healthy and be free of any diseases. Ensuring good nutrition is a way to make sure that our kids are healthy and that most likely means that the kids are getting adequate and balanced nutrition. In this book, we will present 10 signs of good nutrition to make sure that your kids are getting balanced and complete nutrition.

The first way to gauge whether a kid is getting the food he or she needs is to measure their height and weight and see if they match the average for that age. Moreover, we must check with the pediatrician to make sure that the height and weight are fine since our comparisons may be flawed. It is always good to track the child's height and weight to see how well they are doing.

Strong bones are a good sign that your child is getting the good nutrition that they need. Giving them a lot of milk and other related foods is a good way to ensure that, since they contain calcium, it is very good for young, growing children.

Healthy skin is a sign of good nutrition too. Foods that are a source of Vitamin A are very good for the skin. They include vegetables such as carrots, sweet potatoes, and broccoli, and fruits such as papaya, peaches, and mangoes. To maintain good skin, it is also important that sunscreen is applied before going out in the sun.

Below are many other signs that shows that your child has good nutrition:

Having good vision is another sign of good nutrition. For this, you should always allow kids to wear sunglasses in the sun, get their eye sight checked every year, or visit the pediatrician.

Having adequate muscle development is a sign that your child is getting good nutrition and exercising properly. Apart from a good diet, it is also good that your child plays games to be active.

Healthy teeth are another sign that your child is getting the nutrition they need. Vitamin D and calcium are important for maintaining healthy teeth.

Shiny hair is also a sign that your children are getting adequate nutrition. Seafood such as salmon and tuna are a source of nutrients such as Omega 3s which are good for hair.

Strong fingernails are yet another sign of good nutrition.

Your child should be getting 8 hours of sleep and should be sleeping soundly

Finally, an active child is a child who is getting good nutrition.

Not only are adults risking becoming overweight, getting heart disease, or any other disease for that matter; even children are at risk for things like this as well. With this reality, parents need to be more aware of their kids' nutrition. One of the best ways to deal with such a reality is to prevent it from happening to your kids. One of your best bets for combating these things is exercise and a healthy, balanced diet that contains the right nutrition. It's never too early to be aware and start your children on good nutrition, and it will be a good practice that they can carry on to adulthood and benefit from it even in the long run.

Good nutrition can start even before your child takes in solid foods. You can practice this by opting for breast milk over formula. It is the purest and most natural source of nutrients for an infant. It contains high sources of bacteria-fighting components to help your child keep away from sickness; other than this, it also has the necessary nutrients to help your child develop mentally and physically. As your child grows, you can continue to practice good nutrition by being careful with the foods that you introduce. Instead of having your young one eat instant baby food, try boiling and mashing real foods such as potatoes, sweet potatoes, peas, and carrots. Many toddlers can be prone to food allergies, so make it a point to introduce new foods one at a time. Keep foods such as eggs and nuts for when your child is older since these are common allergy foods. Avoid foods with high sodium and sugar content.

By the time that your kids reach school age, they will have grown accustomed to eating nutritious foods, but this may not necessarily mean that they will not be picky. Sometimes as kids grow older, then it becomes more difficult to feed them. If you have a picky eater, try serving different kinds of dishes so that they don't grow tired of foods easily. Try not to make a big deal over them, not eating all of their vegetables or other food. Instead, try to supplement the lost nutrients with healthy snacks that have the same nutritional value. Do make it a point to introduce as many different kinds of food possible to your kid. A well rounded palate will mean that your kids will be more open to eating different dishes that contain different nutrients.

Raising healthy, happy children is the most important and challenging job in the world. Parents have a lot of things to think about when it comes to the health of their children. Today, the sad fact is that our children are becoming less healthy, even though they have some of the best health and fitness resources available. Sedentary lifestyles and poor nutritional choices by parents have contributed to the fact that kids today just aren't as healthy as they could, or should be.

Putting the Pieces Together

To have healthy children, you need to make sure that they have the right balance of diet and physical activity every day. Many parents work long hours and find it difficult to get their kids interested in physical exercise and eating right. But even if you work a lot and aren't able to spend as much time with your kids as you might like, you can still take some simple steps to instill healthy habits into their routines. Kids look up to parents and emulate their actions. Taking steps to improve your health can be a major step forward in the journey toward raising healthy children. Finding the balance is going to take time, as well as trial and error. But as your child grows and you get to understand them more, this should come easier to you as you progress.

Exercise for Kids

Kids need to get plenty of physical activity every day. Some parents get enthusiastic about exercise and try to introduce regular fitness routines for their kids to follow. This isn't always a bad thing, but parents need to remember that healthy children are happy kids and kids are the happiest when they are having fun. When fitness becomes a chore, kids will do whatever they can to avoid it. Parents should try to find fun, interesting ways for their kids to exercise.

For some kids, joining a sports team or taking a fitness-based class, like karate or ballet, is a great way to get exercise. If your child likes sports and social activities, signing him or her up for a team or class may be just the ticket to increase physical activity. Not all kids enjoy organized sports, so parents will need to work a little harder to find physical activities for kids with other interests. Taking family hikes, going for bicycle rides, or long walks can be great forms of exercise for kids who don't want to be involved with structured sports or exercise programs.

The important thing is to get kids physically moving. Raising healthy children requires parents to be sure that their kids are getting some physical activity regularly.

Parents needs to work with their children to find fun and engaging activities for the long haul. Emphasizing this to your children is also crucial.

Nutrition for Kids

One of the biggest challenges parents face in getting their kids to eat healthy foods is the fact that kids are naturally attracted to junk food, so parents need to take action to get their kids to eat healthier. Like the rest of us, kids need to have plenty of fruits, vegetables, fiber, essential fats, and lean protein to stay healthy and strong.

Parents often lose the battle for a healthy diet with their kids by being too strict when it comes to eating plans. Don't be overly restrictive with your child's diet. Just like exercise, when kids, perceive that they are being forced to behave in a certain way, they are likely to rebel the first chance they get.

Make Healthy Eating Fun

You buy the groceries, so you probably have a good idea of what your kids like to eat. Take some time to make a list of the healthier foods they enjoy. For example, if your child eats a lot of junk food, but likes a particular vegetable, try finding similar vegetables to introduce into their diet. Many kids will begin to enjoy food after they have tried it a few times. Whatever you do, don't make healthy eating into a contest of the wills. If kids know that they are going to be in for an argument at every meal, they'll never enjoy eating healthy foods.

Sneaking in the Good Stuff

With some kids, you can't win when it comes to food. Some will not eat vegetables, no matter how much mom and dad threaten, beg, plead, or scream. This can be a big challenge for parents, but there are sneaky ways to add good, nutritious foods into the diets of die-hard junk food fans. For example, parents can use a food processor to liquefy fruits and vegetables and sneak them into a child's meal. This tactic won't work well with older kids, but it can be a way to get some fruits and vegetables into the system of young children.

Educate Your Kids About Healthy Foods

It's important to educate them about the importance of eating right and exercising if you want to raise healthy children. Parents shouldn't have to spend all their time sneaking nutritious foods into their kids' meals. Educated kids understand how what they eat and how much they exercise affects the quality of life that they will have as adults.

The most important fact of all in raising healthy children is to be a good example. Remember that your kids learn about life through what they see you do. If you've been getting on by takeout and junk food, start taking steps to clean up your diet. If your kids see you eating healthy and exercising, they'll be more likely to do it themselves.

And just as kids take vitamins to make up for deficiencies in their everyday diet, parents need to add supplements to their diets to give them what they need. Try adding a healthy protein supplement like Profect - a liquid shot from Protica - to your diet to make sure you are getting enough protein. Remember that healthy children usually have healthy parents, so take the time to take care of yourself. Your kids will thank you for it.

Top Tips for Healthy Kid Nutrition

Unhealthy diets have been related to many problems for children ranging from growth abnormalities to learning and behavioural problems at school. A child's diet also sets them up for life as an adult, often with any problems caused by a bad childhood diet only becoming evident when they grow older. If you follow these five steps you will be helping to give your kid the best possible start in life. This is particularly important because it is not just their childhood that will be affected by what they eat when they are young.

Firstly it's important to realise that since children are growing their nutritional and calorific needs are different from yours as an adult, in fact children under the age of 5 have very different needs compared to adults. A child under

5 will need a diet that includes foods with higher fat content than an adult and they should avoid calorie restricted or high fiber (such as whole grain) diets. From the age of 5, a gradual transition to a more 'adult like' diet can be taken with lower fat foods and more whole grain.

1. A suitable diet for kids should be varied

A kid's diet should be varied and should include a selection of foods from all the 5 food groups, this will make sure that they get all the nutrients that they need. The five food groups include:

Starchy foods - for example bread, cereals, potatoes, rice, pasta. These foods should make up a large part of a child's diet and children should be encouraged to eat foods from this group.

Fruit and vegetables - fresh, tinned, frozen and dried fruit and vegetables. To encourage children to like these types of food they should be given 4-5 servings from as wide a range as possible each day.

Dairy foods - milk, yogurt, cheese. Around one pint of milk, 125g of yogurt or 30g of cheese a day is a healthy amount of dairy products for a child to consume. Children under the age of 5 should not have fat reduced milk such as semi skimmed milk, while children over five can move onto fat reduced varieties.

Meat and proteins - meat, poultry, fish, eggs, beans, lentils, nuts. Children should eat 2 or 3 portions a day.

Fatty and Sugary foods - while fats can be a useful source of energy for children under 5, foods which provide some nutritional value as well as fat should be chosen, for example milk, lean meat, oilyfish, cheese and yogurt rather than cake, crisps, chocolate and pastry.

If you choose a good mix of foods from the categories described above this will help make sure that your kid is getting many of the vitamins and minerals they need for good health. However surveys carried out by the Food Standards Agency and the Department of Health suggest that many children don't get enough of a large range of vitamins and minerals including vitamin D, vitamin A, potassium, calcium, phosphorus and iron.

Furthermore, the same research also suggests that children tend to get too much salt, fat, sugar and saturated fat in their diets, this is particularly a problem for teenagers who have more control over their own diets and needless to say, they tend not to eat what is good for them.

2. Check your kids' daily Calorific intake

These government figures are guides for the daily requirements of children, as they are guides they may vary from one child to another. An active child will need more calories than an inactive one, even for the same child their calorific intake may be higher on one day and lower the next.

If a child regularly exceeds these guidelines, they may become over weight (obese), this is a growing problem in many parts of the developed world, for children and adults alike.

Calories per day by age:

years - boys - girls

1-3 - 1,230 - 1,165

4-6 - 1,715 - 1,545

7-10 - 1,970 - 1,740

11-14 - 2,220 - 1,845

15-18 - 2,755 - 2,110

Adults - 2,550 - 1,940

Calorie requirement per day adapted from NHS choices

3. Check your kids salt intake

Research suggests that a large intake of salt in adults can cause high blood pressure. While high blood pressure in children is unusual it's also unlikely to be healthy for children to have too much salt. While adults should have no more than 6g of salt per day, children should have even less.

It's important to avoid adding salt when cooking or eating meals and foods high in salt should also be avoided. This includes foods such as crisps, sauces, processed foods and many ready meals. Unfortunately salt is often used as a flavour enhancer and so is widely used in the food manufacturing industry, even for food specifically for children.

1-3 years - 2g a day (0.8g sodium)
4-6 years - 3g a day (1.2g sodium)
7-10 years - 5g a day (2g sodium)
11 years upward - 6g a day (2.5g sodium)

*Recommended levels of salt for children (1g of salt corresponds to 0.4g of sodium)

4. Check your kids' diet includes a source of Vitamin D

Recent research has suggested that many children may be deficient in Vitamin D, particularly in winter as the main source of vitamin D is from the action of sun on our skin. Vitamin D is found in a few natural foods such as oily fish (sardine, salmon, mackerel, pilchard and tuna) and a few foods are fortified with small amounts of Vitamin D (infant formula milk, margarine and some breakfast cereals).

However during winter when sunlight levels are low the main source of Vitamin D is supplements and, in fact, the government recommends that some children take vitamin D as a matter of course, either prescribed or over-the-counter from pharmacies, health food shops and the Internet.

5. Check to ensure that your kids' diet includes sources of Iron rich foods

It is important to include iron rich food in a child's diet, as iron enables blood to carry oxygen around the body. Low levels of iron can particularly be a problem for vegetarians as it is more difficult to absorb iron form fruit and vegetables, although adding vitamin C can help with absorption (for example having baked beans with sliced tomatoes).

> Excellent - liver and kidney
> Very Good - wheat germ bread, dried fruit, beef, pilchard, sardines
> Good - whole meal bread, pulses, lentils, beans, lamb, pork, vegetable, fish (including fishfingers)

SNACKS FOR KIDS AND WEIGHTLOSS

Snacking has become a feature in the routine of most families every day. Due to the fact that finding time for a healthy meal is a difficult task, snacking has become a major feature in most of our diets. It is essential to keep ontop of snacks, and also make sure that what we do consume between regular mealtimes is healthy and good for our bodies. Of course, this is also true when it comes to our children, and ensuring their health and well-being can be an even trickier task. Kids bodies need sources of energy to keep them active, and to help them grow and develop into adolescence and adulthood. Additionally, with the increasing problem of obesity in children, it is essential to ensure your child has only the best of healthy snacks throughout the day.

The first consideration to take into account is your child's happiness. Achieving a balance between healthy living and a happy child is something many parents adopting the gung-ho 'my way or no way' approach fail to reach. Not only is this antiquated parenting, but it is also a sure-fire way to turn your child off healthy living. Don't completely ban treats, but keep them to a minimum. Think of everything in balance and moderation as the best way to achieve a healthy diet.

A good place to start is with introducing fruit and vegetables. Experts tell us that we should consume a minimum of five portions daily, and this might at first seem like a high hurdle to meet. However, by introducing vegetables into every meal, and promoting fruit as the alternative choice between times, you can sneak in those added portions, and they really do add up. It's also a good idea to maintain an open mind yourself, and to experiment with other fruits and vegetables until you find something appealing to your child's taste-buds. After a while, fruit and vegetables will become an engrained part of daily life, and will be something your children crave at every opportunity. Until that point however, it is best to take a sensible approach to your child's healthy eating plan.

Healthy eating is a scary phrase for most adults, and for children, it can be even more daunting. It's up to you as the parent to enforce healthy eating through making sensible life choices, and it's also important to ensure your child understands the need for a healthy balanced lifestyle.

Healthy snacks for kids are important to provide more nutrition and energy for them. Children need a lot of good nutrition to develop and to get them through each day, especially at school.

Children's foods are normally not enough for the energy they need and they require healthy snacks to give them the extra energy to keep growing.

Every time they eat any meals or snacks, it should be an opportunity to give children more nutrition, which they always need to help them to think better, and concentrate for longer. Missing out on these opportunities can lead to worse social interactions, and poor grades in school.

Always try to limit junk food as that gives them empty calories and contributes to restlessness and lack of concentration. Fast foods and junk foods contain loads of fat, calories, sugar and salt and do not add much to the amount of nutrition they need to help them focus. Otherwise, you will have their stomachs filled-up of nothing!

You see, children raised on healthy eating habits do not have a problem really with healthy snacks. Why?

Because that's how they were raised!

Some kids have no problem eating vegetables, salads, fruits and other healthy snacks for kids. In fact, they love them to bits. And they might only be two years old.

Some, on the other hand, of about seven years of age; may have no problem eating whatever healthy food is prepared for them.

However, they are able to eat them easily without stressing.

If a parent has a high cholesterol level for instance; their cholesterol level would have for the most part, probably come from how they're eating and food choices. What do you think they'll pass on to their children?

No, not cholesterol; but the lifestyle they have lived in terms of diet and how they've cooked! This sets your child up for disaster before they even get the opportunity to create healthy habits for themselves.

If your children grow up seeing you eating fast food mostly and eating out all the time. They'll tend to do exactly the same as they saw and learnt while growing up.

It is imperative to teach our kids the importance and significance of nutrition in their lives and yours, as this is what they will build upon for their future.

Don't worry if you haven't been preparing the right foods and healthy enough meals for your kids to eat; the time to start is NOW. Better late than never. You can begin to talk about it to them. It'll sink in with time.

But you must be persistent and take control. You can indulge them sometimes and you can give them some foods not tremendously healthy, but those should be the minority. Set the example to eat healthy, and in time, you will see the positive side effects that this has for their future! The most important thing is that they should be getting good nutrition in their main meals and that their meals are balanced the majority of the time.

Don't over-indulge them. That's the mistake some of us parents make. Sometimes we feel guilty for other things, and then give them unhealthy, sugary and fatty snacks instead to try to make up for it. Wrong choice. This shows that when bad things happen, the reward is to eat unhealthily.

If this is something you do as a lifestyle, it could backfire health-wise for them, and you're not actually doing things in their best interests.

Make smart choices when it comes to getting healthy snacks for kids, and the decision will payoff for them and for you big time. They need these in their diet for extra nutrition and energy to grow big and strong.

Parents everywhere face the dilemma of attempting to get kids to eat healthier snacks. Sometimes convincing a child to eat healthy snacks is not as easy as it is made out to be. While parents are wise in their effort to try and get children to consume healthier foods, kids will argue that sweet treats and "bad-for-you" goodies taste better than healthy foods offered. So, how does a parent convince a child to eat healthier snacks throughout the day?

One way to ensure that children eat healthy snacks is to give them super healthy foods from the outset. The sooner parents introduce their children to healthy snacks, the better. If a child eats healthy snacks all their life and knows nothing else, the child is less likely to give parents a hassle when parents choose to introduce new, healthy foods into the child's regular diet.

Parents looking to encourage their children to eat super healthy foods should make snack time fun. When kids are having fun, they focus on enjoying the time they are having and there is less focus on the fact that they are trying something new. There are plenty of ways to make snacks, both fun and healthy too. Let's take a look at a few fun snacks kids tend to enjoy.

The beverage you give your child during snack time or mealtime is just as important as the foods selected. Instead of offering cola or kool-aid and sugar-filled beverages, offer a child a glass of milk or a glass of juice instead. While juice has sugar in it, the fruit juice will still carry more vitamins and minerals than kool-aid offers. The juice selections can also be frozen as well, thereby giving a child a super tasty treat.

Yogurt is an excellent snack for children and is better than pudding from pudding packs. You can even give your child granola chips to add ontop of the yogurt, and yogurt is just as delicious with dried fruits, nuts, and banana chips on top. Since yogurts are offered in a variety of flavors, parents will have no trouble finding yogurts that their kids love.

Parents should opt for fresh fruits whenever possible rather than give kids a fruit cocktail that is fixed in heavy syrup. Cutting up some watermelon, honeydew, and cantaloupe makes for a perfect midday snack. Strawberries mixed with fresh raspberries and blueberries are also an excellent option. The latter berries can be quickly put in a blender with some ice for a super cool and refreshing snack for kids.

Cereal snacks are a great way for parents to offer children snack diversity. Choosing healthy cereals like Cheerios (TM) and puffed rice are better cereal selections than those coated with sugar and loaded with calories. The healthy cereal can be mixed with dried fruits like apricots, bananas, and the like, and granola helps make this type of snack a hearty treat for children.

In the growing up phase, while teaching your kids the right habits and manners, eating habits often stay neglected. A child tends to pick up an extra snack anytime during the day between their regular meals. These snacks, if planned properly, can add to their nutrition and energy value. But if not, it can lead to grave problems, like child obesity.

In the fast-paced life, children often pick up cookies, chips, doughnuts, and colas with their pocket money. While a little of these things help him/ her to get adjusted to outside food, a greater intake of these foods could result in health issues, including liver malfunction and other digestive system problems. Obesity or overly lean frame is the only aftermath. Therefore, it is the parent's responsibility to keep a check on the snack habits of their kids and see to the fact that whatever they eat in off-time snacks should not be crossing approximately 150 calories.

If you find it very difficult to restrict your kid's snack habit, then the alternate way of keeping the calories in check is to check the contents of their plate. A diet full of fiber and proteins will keep them full and reduce their cravings for unhealthy food. You can gradually develop their snack habits around fruits like apples, oranges, and pears. Introduce cereal bars, baked chips, low-fat chips, yogurt, and popcorn in their snack plate. These foods will satisfy their cravings for tasty, trendy foods while keeping them fit and fine.

A good place to start is by introducing fruit and vegetables. Experts tell us that we should consume a minimum of five portions daily, and this might at first seem like a high hurdle to meet. However, by introducing vegetables into every meal, and promoting fruit as the choice between times, you can sneak in those added portions, and they add up. It's also a good idea to maintain an open mind yourself and experiment with other fruits and vegetables until you find something appealing to your child's taste buds. After a while, fruit and vegetables will become an ingrained part of daily life and be something your children crave at every opportunity. Until that point, however, it is best to take a sensible approach to your child's healthy eating plan.

A snack can contribute to extra energy for your kids. Afternoon snacks gives them extra energy after school. It helps them to concentrate on their homework. However, not all snacks are healthy for them. You have to select a healthy snack for them.

As a mother or father, you have to be able to provide them a healthy snack. You could prepare it yourself to make it fresh. What healthy snacks can you prepare?

Children love anything they can dip. You can prepare it using low-fat ingredients or make nutritious hummus, salsa, or bean dip. Your children will also like whole wheat crackers, pita triangles, or chips with tortilla baked. Perfect dips from fruit include applesauce, flavored yogurt, sourcream with low fat which is sweetened by brown sugar or honey and topping from caramel ice cream.

Most kids are snackers, more then they are meal eaters. It isn't uncommon for kids to want to graze versus sitting down to the table to eat an actual meal. While mealtime is important and should become a family habit, snacks will be inevitable. Helping your children to learn healthy snacking habits can help them maintain a healthy weight throughout their lives. Follow these tips to ensure healthy snacking patterns with your children.

Let your kids help you with the shopping list. Ask them what kinds of products they'd like for their snacks. When kids have a say in what they are eating, they will be more likely to eat it. Help them get excited about different choices.

Be sure your kids know where the healthy snacks are kept. If they know how to find the product easily, and they know how to prepare it if needed, the chance of them eating it is a lot higher.

Prepare your fruit and vegetables and put them in see-through containers in the fridge, so your kids know where they are and can easily access them. Having these fat burning foods on hand will be great for your diet as well.

Keep fresh fruit on the counter. Explain to your kids when the fruit is ripe and best to eat. The more they know, the more likely they are to partake.

Pre-portion out snacks, such as nuts or whole-grain crackers, for your kids in plastic bags or small see-through containers. This will help to avoid mindless eating, overeating, and overdoing it on the snacks.

Avoid buying too many sweets and sugary snacks. Keep them higher on shelves if you do buy them, so they are not as readily available to your kids. If the lower shelves contain healthier snack options, they will be more likely to reach for those foods.

These small practices can help get your kids into good habits of healthy eating and keep them feeling great.

Children, perhaps more so than adults, need snacks. The eating habits of a child typically mirror those of their parents/caregiver, consisting of three daily meals: breakfast, lunch, and dinner. However, as most parents/caregivers can attest, getting a child to clean their plate can be challenging.

Anxiousness, coupled with a proportionately small stomach, make it difficult for children to sit down and eat an entire meal. As a result, children may not receive enough calories each day. This is unhealthy for both children and adults because fewer calories mean less energy and nutrients to fuel the body and protect it from foreign objects, like viruses and bacteria. Preparing small, nutritious snacks will help children consume the calories they need for energy and the nutrients they need to stay healthy.

Heart Healthy Whole Grains

Whole grains are building blocks for a nutritious and filling snack. Parents must take caution, though. Most "whole grain" foods are made using only a small portion of actual whole grains. Also, whole grain cereals and snack bars are often over-processed and rich in sugar. The best whole grain snacks include oatmeal, topped with fresh blueberries, or a small portion of brown rice and vegetables. While the portions may be small (two children sharing a single bowl of oatmeal, for example), the nutritious advantage is huge. Whole grains are associated with a lessened risk of heart disease, and they are a fundamental source of energy!

Delicious Dairy Products

Dairy products make the perfect mid-day snack for children. Foods like low-fat cheese sticks, yogurt, and cottage cheese with fresh fruit offer two main nutritional benefits. First, they are a good source of protein. Second, they have moderate amounts of unsaturated fat. Studies show that replacing ordinary fat with unsaturated fat, like that found in dairy products, reduces the amount of bad cholesterol (low-density lipoprotein) in your blood (i). Although cholesterol worries are something we typically associate with adults, children can also benefit from eating foods that keep LDL levels low.

Organic Fruits and Vegetables

Organic fruits and vegetables make the best snacks for children. The fruit is a good early morning snack because it is a good source of carbohydrates, water, and vitamins to sustain energy throughout the day. Apples, peaches, grapes, oranges, and watermelon are all great choices. When it comes to late afternoon snacks, though, vegetables are the way to go. Vegetables contain fewer carbohydrates yet are rich in minerals. Serving snacks like raw broccoli, carrots, sliced tomatoes, and celery can replenish a child's nutrient levels without overfilling their stomachs before dinner. To make things more fun, serve a low-fat side to add some extra flavor to the vegetables. Low fat ranch dip, balsamic vinegar and olive oil, light seasoning, or all-natural organic peanut butter complement vegetables in a delicious way. Also, dipping is fun! The more fun a snack or meal is, the more likely a child will eat the entire portion.

Healthy whole grains, dairy products, fruit, and raw vegetables are hands down the best snacks for kids. They offer a moderate serving of calories, healthy fat, protein, and plenty of vitamins and minerals. Holistic dentistry holds that overall health is reflected in the mouth; following these snack guidelines will keep your child's body healthy, and their mouths cavity-free.

Obesity is becoming a major problem among kids today. As a parent, it is important to help your child lead a healthy lifestyle. Below is a list of healthy snacks you can quickly and easily prepare for your children.

Top Healthy Snacks for Kids

Whether they're running, jumping, chasing, playing, dancing or just following you around asking questions, one thing is for certain - kids are always on the move! And all of that energy leads to large appetites.

But when it comes to getting kids to eat healthy snacks to renew that energy, many parents find themselves stuck in gridlock. So how can parents compete with endless junk food options and get their kids to eat healthier snacks? You can start by offering these top ten healthy snacks that will get your kids excited about eating right.

Ants on a Log

This fun and healthy snack for kids is a classic that's been pleasing youthful palates for generations. All you need is some celery stalks, peanut butter, and raisins. Simply slice celery stalksdown the middle and spread each side with peanut butter. Next, place raisins on top of the peanut butter, spacing them out to look like ants marching on a log.

Homemade Snack Mix

Snack mixes are great on-the-go snacks for kids. They can also be an excellent healthy snack, depending on what's in them. Making your own snack mix is an inexpensive and easy alternative to buying store-bought mixes. Use ingredients likenuts, dried fruit chips, seeds, granola, and carob for a healthy and delicious snack kids will love.

Green Bean Chips

A healthier alternative to potato chips, green bean chips make eating green beans fun again! Kids will love the crunchy, salty flavor. They can usually be found at your local health food store. Many regular grocery stores are also starting to carry them too so be sure to check out using this healthier snack to replace regular potato chips.

Hummus and Pita Slices

Made from fiber and protein packed chickpeas, hummus is a delicious and versatile spread. It comes in a variety of flavors and is available at most grocery stores. It's also simple to make from scratch at home. Serve with toasted pita slices for a yummy snack kids can get excited about.

Sunflower Seeds

Sunflower seeds are another fun and healthy snack for kids. They're a great source of vitamin E and a good source of vitamins B1 and B6 too. Shelled or unshelled, roasted, salted or not, your kids are sure to enjoy this classic healthy snack. For a fun family activity, grow some sunflowers in the yard or in pots and have your kids help you harvest them.

Cinnamon Toast

This snack combines cinnamon, bread, margarine, and a touch of sugar - all things kids love! Simply toast your favorite healthy bread choice, spread lightly with margarine and sprinkle with a touch of sugar and cinnamon. Your kids will be requesting more of this favorite low-fat snack.

Popcorn Made Healthy

Popcorn isn't as unhealthy as everyone thinks it is. It's actually all of the stuff we put on it that makes it so bad for us. Kids love popcorn, but all that butter and salt equals a bad snack choice. Make popcorn healthy again by popping it plain and topping it with nutritional yeast, which tastes great and is full of amino acids and B complex vitamins.

Yoghurt and Pretzels

Calcium is essential for healthy bones and teeth and yogurt is rich in calcium, not to mention cultures that aid in digestive tract health. Yogurt comes in all kinds of fun flavors that mimic the taste of your kid's favorite desserts. You can also buy plain yogurt in bulk and top it with fresh fruits. Add some pretzel sticks for a great healthy snack.

Avocado

Fat is actually a good part of any diet, as long as it's the right kind of fat. Avocados are full of healthy unsaturated fats. They're also a great source of potassium, fiber, and vitamin C. Mash up with tomato and a splash of lime for homemade guacamole, use instead of mayo on a sandwich, or place on toasted bread for a quick, nutritious snack.

Smoothies

A smoothie is a lot like a milkshake-only much healthier! Your kids will love the fruity ice-cream like taste and you can sneak in all kinds of healthy additions. Use fresh fruit like strawberries and bananas, soy or rice-milk and limit the sugar. You can also use smoothies as a way to introduce new fruits for your kids to enjoy like mangoes and kiwi.

These healthy snacks for kids are sure to get your kids more excited about eating right.

HEALTHY LIFESTYLE FOR KIDS

A healthy lifestyle for kids is extremely important and it involves making the time needed to prepare healthy meals for your children. If left to their own devices we all know what a child's menu would consist of, and any child who controls his or her own diet by zapping favorite foods in the microwave is in for trouble.

While it is the parents' responsibility to ensure a healthy lifestyle for kids; research has shown that there are several external factors that are also responsible for our overweight children. Fast food is the number one culprit with their high calorie content and portion size. More children are being driven to school instead of good old fashioned 'walking the two blocks to school' concept. Of course this can also be attributed to child safety concerns. With the advent of the television, videogame console and the computer it has become increasingly difficult to pry a child away and get them outdoors to play. Ask your child to stop playing their videogame and come outside for a game of one-on-one basketball; the look you will get is as good as asking whether you are from outer space! Our assignment as parents is to make sure our children know the values and limitations of this new technology, and when to step away from the computer and on to the playground.

Camps are an excellent solution for tackling this problem; they are geared to provide nutritious food and a whole lot of interesting activities that keep kids active and on their toes. It is hoped that the right eating habits and healthy lifestyle for kids taught at camp will translate to the home environment as well. Some of the benefits of sending your child to camp regularly can be summed up as:

- Camps are designed to reinforce positive development of children.
- At camp the child learns about foods that are good for them; these choices are presented in a fun environment in the company of other children, making it an overall happier experience to eat the things that are good for you but you may not like.
- Camps have adult staff who serve as mentors to support healthy behavior in terms of eating and activities.

- There is a range of healthy outdoor activities even for the most die hard television fans and it is always fun to get involved in activities with other children.

At camp children experience learning made fun through group activities that stimulate and educate; best of all there is a firm emphasis on the value of good nutrition.

Your child will learn valuable social skills when it comes to talking about their health and nutrition.

With technologies continually rising, almost every activity in modern life is connected with the Internet, gadgetry, and other computer-age advancements. But are the days of activity and sweat-breaking exercise for kids lost in today's fast-paced life? Fitness and kids can still come together, despite all the high-tech toys. How can we make sure that kids understand why they need fitness and help them learn to enjoy it?

Is there a need for exercise for kids?

Being overweight or obese is no longer confined to adults and old age. In the US alone, 1 out of 3 children is either overweight or obese. And this ratio is increasing at an alarming rate every year. This percentage can be accounted to the shortage or total loss of effective fitness and kids programs.

The weight problems kids are facing as youth will affect them not only now, but as they grow into adulthood. They will continue to suffer from adverse health, poor self-image, and obesity issues. However, if parents and guardians could teach children enjoyable exercises now, then their lives, both physiologically and socially, can still be saved.

Can fitness and kids still mesh together?

It is possible to teach kids a love for fitness if it is approached in the right way. As a parent or guardian, you must understand the value of fitness for yourself, so you can easily introduce the appropriate physical health program to your children. First of all, fitness is not merely a set of exercises. You must include proper diet, hygiene, and emotional health in their daily lives. Fitness and healthy living must become a lifestyle

Fitness and kids can easily work together if there is a fun factor. Explain to them the benefits of each activity as you introduce them. Start by being an example and encourage your children to join in. Soon you will have a fun, family-fitting program where you will be building healthy bodies and a great relationship!

How to get started with your fitness and kids program?

Indulge in outdoor activities. When was the last time you and the kids went to the park? Revive the thrill of camping trips, hiking, biking, and other similar adventures. Make it a habit to run together, play jump rope and boxing, and being involved in interactive sports at least twice a week.

Give your family diet a makeover, with the kids' help. Let them help plan healthy foods and make sure you incorporate their choices. Ensure that fruits, vegetables, and other nutritious sources are part of your daily diet and teach your kids why they are important.

Most of the values, habits, routines, and attitudes we have as adults began when we were still children. If you have a positive outlook on life, you will likely be raised in an environment that values optimism. If you are thrifty, you were probably taught how to be a smart spender as a child. If you are a responsible worker, you probably took after your parents whom you have always seen as such hardworking people.

However, you may employ some techniques to encourage your kid to eat their veggies. One way to do this is to make their veggies look fun and exciting. Combine different colors and use these veggies to create playful shapes that would entice them to munch on these treats.

Another way would be to disguise the vegetables or fruits like turning it into juice, smoothie, or shake. Moreover, you may also give incentives and rewards occasionally to reinforce your kid's healthy eating habits.

1. Establish a healthy sleep routine for your kid

Sleep is an essential part of one's health. Some kids would always stay up late watching television or playing video games. This act is not a healthy habit. While the immediate effects of sleeping late are not evident, the long term effects of a lack of sleep can have on a person are extremely dangerous. Draft a schedule for their naptime and night sleeping time.

Also, make sure they wake up early in the morning. It is not a good idea to let your kid oversleep. As the adage goes, "Early to bed, early to rising makes one healthy, wealthy and wise!"

2. Allow your kid to play outside.

Physical activity is important to hone several skills such as fine and gross motor skills, muscle strength, flexibility, endurance, stamina, and so on. By playing outside, your kid will be able to get all the necessary exercise they need to thrive and develop properly.

3. Set a good example.

Observational learning is indeed one of the most effective ways to teach a child. Because of this, you need to ensure that you set a good example and practice what you preach so that it is easier for your child to take on healthy habits such as sleeping early, exercising, and eating healthy.

It's not "cool" to be fat, but that has not prevented an obesity epidemic from occurring among American youth. Childhood obesity increased from 5 percent in 1964 to about 13 percent in 1994. Today, it is about 20 percent - and rising. Children spend an excessive amount of time watching television, using the computer, and playing video games. All these activities are partly to be blamed for this escalating rate. They spend upto five to six hours a day involved in these sedentary activities. Perhaps it wouldn't matter if they were sufficiently active at other times, but most of them aren't.

To make matters worse, children are bombarded with well-crafted TV ads from fast-food chains and other purveyors of high-fat, high-sugar meals and snacks. A recent study reported that children aged two to six that watch television are more likely to choose food products advertised on TV than children who do not watch such commercials. These highly effective advertising campaigns, combined with a physically inactive lifestyle, have produced a generation of kids who are at high risk for obesity-associated medical conditions.

The major health threat in the early development of Type II diabetes (adult-onset), particularly in children with a family history of the disease. Doctors are reporting a surge in young adolescents developing Type II diabetes - which can lead to heart and kidney disease, high blood pressure, stroke, limb amputations, and blindness. People who develop diabetes in adolescence face a diminished quality of life and shortened life span, particularly if the disease progresses untreated. It's a scary prospect for our children, but, in many cases, obesity and diabetes are preventable.

Parents should be involved in their kids' daily physical activities. In today's educational system, most schools offer PE (Physical Education) classes that allow kids to participate in physical activities and help them be more active. They also allow them to interact with their classmates on another level. However, these PE classes are not enough to help with their daily activity allowance. Many of these classes have been cut or reduced in recent years because of a lack of funding.

Physical education should be a top priority; after-school extra-curricular activities and sports are also vital. Children must develop a lifestyle that includes regular exercise, as well as a healthy diet. Parents need to set limit on the time their children are engaged in passive activities. Pediatricians recommend restricting children to one to two hours per day on TV and computers combined, unless, of course, they are Internet hackers - but there are always exceptions to the rule.

Fortunately, some schools now provide meals that are lower in fat and include healthy helpings of fruits and vegetables. Parental involvement remains the most important key to our children's healthy diets. Programs to educate parents about nutrition are essential. Fast food should be banned from all schools. Period!

For many, the fast-food industry is of great help. It offers parents an easy solution when dinner can't be prepared due to time restrictions. With hectic daily schedules, it is becoming difficult for parents to cook healthy meals for their kids. Therefore, they seek the easy way out unwittingly poisoning their kids while eating at a fast-food chain. Changing eating habits and lifestyles is not easy, but the health benefits for children are a wonderful payoff for parents willing to take on the task. Important things parents can do to curtail the obesity epidemic among children:

Limit TV viewing and time on the computer to one to two hours per day. Too much screen time can have adverse effects on a child's development.

Encourage participation in physical activity and sports.

Avoid eating in a fast-food chain. It can become habitual as they are incredibly convenient and cheap, but the effects on a person's health can be monumental in the long run.

Provide nutritious, well-balanced, low-calorie, and low-fat meals.

Limit the availability of high-fat and high-sugar snacks in your home—instead, flavour fruits and vegetables as go-to snacks for your kids.

Make your kids healthy lunches to bring to school. If your kids do get peer pressure from their classmates because of their daily lunchbox, just tell your kids that they are not allergic to fast food but are restricted with the food they can eat.

These are a few possible ways to start making a difference in your kids' health. You will need to focus on feeding them healthy meals and avoid unhealthy snacks. With today's research and development in the food industry, there are many alternatives to snacks that are healthy and taste as good as the unhealthy ones. Chocolate, chips, meals that contain low fat, low cholesterol, and low sugar and help you keep your diet without suffering too much, especially if you have a sweet tooth.

Obesity in Children! This is a true and frightening fact. We will need to face it soon or suffer the consequences. It is a vicious cycle. If parents are obese (overweight), kids tend to follow the same trend. This cycle will have to be interrupted somewhere, and education is the solution. Children need to be taught to develop good eating habits to avoid gaining excess weight. Check with your child's doctor to confirm that his or her obesity isn't due to genetics or some other medical problem (addressed in the first few chapters of the book). Parents can help their children by being supportive. Explain why s/he has to lose weight. Gather family support for him/her. The parent must also be a role model and display good eating habits.

The child needs to grow vertically - not horizontally (due to a large waistline). Don't put them on a strict diet. As mentioned in previous chapters about available diets, it is not recommended to put children through them. These are extreme diets with temporary results. Avoid yo-yo dieting, especially when your child is young. Try maintaining the Food Guide Pyramid of carbohydrates, proteins, fats and oils, and vitamins and minerals. This is necessary for a balanced diet. Reduce the servings of fatty foods. Other foods are also to be consumed in moderation. Remove empty calories from junk food like sweets and snacks. Improvise to give them healthy snacks like milk, fruit, or plain biscuits. Don't eliminate sweets. They'll feel miserable. Limit the amount to be consumed over a week. Slowly replace the sweets with dried fruit to wean their sweet tooth.

Using food to reward a child fosters eating disorders and unhealthy associations with food. They may overeat unnecessarily. Keep a lock on the pantry. Leave healthy snacks readily available on the kitchen counter or inaccessible places in the fridge.

Teach a child to appreciate healthy meals by encouraging involvement in meal preparations. Don't allow them to eat in front of the TV; this creates the bad habit of always eating whenever the television is on.

Teach your child what foods to buy when they're eating outside the home. Kids love fast food. It's common knowledge. However, by slowly reducing their intake of fast food, they eventually eliminate it and gear towards healthy alternatives, such as a veggie burger with vegetables and a salad. Children like variety in their menu. Parents can improvise and invent healthy meals. Emphasize the importance of vegetables, as kids tend to hate greens and stuff themselves with meats. Another trick is to make the child drink a glass of water or milk before the meal. They won't feel hungry since their stomach will be pre-filled with liquid, so they will eat much less to get full.

Exercise together as a family. It promotes bonding, too. Get into some fun activities like roller-blading, biking, or sports. Initially, the persuasion may be tough, but once the ball starts rolling, there's no stopping it.

Set realistic goals for your child to lose weight. Offer loads of praise for goals that are achieved. Keep track of your child's weight and eating habits. Children need guidance to avoid sliding back.

All these efforts can greatly help your child with his/her health issues. Small steps are necessary for successful results. I guess most of you experienced these extreme diets and achieved only temporary results. We all learn from mistakes, and teaching others how to avoid them can be of great help. It will be a long journey for you and your child, but your battle against obesity is halfway won. However, to achieve this victory, we need to take and practice several steps, such as:

Make your children participate in daily school activities and explain to them the importance of being involved with their community. It is vital to get them to participate in these programs so as not to allow unhealthy foods to enter the establishment.

Mandatory PE in each grade level.

The involvement of schools doesn't stop here. Small medical centers should be established to screen students (not for drugs, although sometimes, it can be necessary) for cholesterol or glucose. Below are other food strategies to be considered:

Increase in diabetes, blood pressure, heart disease.

Implementation of prevalence study of school children in the county (3rd and 6th graders) as well as a survey of nutrition optionsin schools (meals and vending).

Measure BMIs (Body Mass Index) in county schools.

With all these ideas in mind, we can finally process the information mentioned above and start realizing that all communities, schools, cities, and governments can be involved in eradicating this terrible disease.

Programs to address cultural differences.

City participation in nutrition and fitness.

Strongly establish public health education in schools so we can influence nutritional and activity/exercise policy.

Tax unhealthy foods to provide subsidy for the sale of fruits, vegetables, whole grains, and beans.

5 Benefits of a Healthy Lifestyle for Kids

With the continuing change that the world is experiencing, more and more children from all over the world are suffering from a case of obesity. This is brought about by the lifestyle change that progress demands. It has never been more important for parents and guardians alike to make sure that their kids have a healthy lifestyle. Obesity, if not addressed can cause serious health problems in childhood and later in life. Children will benefit physically, mentally, socially and academically from a healthy lifestyle of proper nutrition and exercise.

But what benefits exactly does a healthy living have on children? What good does a healthy lifestyle give? There are plenty of benefits a healthy lifestyle offers, but here I will be mentioning five.

1. A child who eats right and exercises regularly will have a physically healthy body that can lower risk from high blood pressure, high cholesterol, diabetes and more. These conditions are usually associated with obesity.
2. Aside from physical health, a healthy lifestyle will also provide improved mental health. Proper diet

and exercise helps children handle mental challenges well. A healthy lifestyle provides better sleep at night and more energy to make children feel better mentally. It can also lessen depression.

3. Healthy kids also benefit socially. Physically active and healthy kids usually have high self-esteem, which will help them, make friends. Kids who join sports or other physical activities are more likely to make friends than to stay in front of the TV and computer.

4. Healthy kids are also more likely to benefit emotionally. They'll have high self-esteem because they feel better about their appearance physically. They'll also be more confident in themselves in socializing with other children. Developing early-onset confidence does wonders for a child as they age and get placed into various social situations.

5. Lastly, kids who have a healthy lifestyle benefit academically. Children who eat properly, exercise regularly, and get ample sleep have the physical and mental energy to deal with academic challenges daily. They are also able to retain their lessons better than kids who have an unhealthy lifestyle.

These are just some of the benefits that children who have a healthy lifestyle experience. It's important for parents and guardians to monitor and guide their children to live healthy. If not addressed properly, children will suffer serious health problems because of obesity. As they say, prevention is always better than the cure. So a child who is healthy will live a better life than those who are not.

DIFFERENT GAMES AND ACTIVITIES FOR KIDS

There are different kinds of great games on the market today that are available for children in a wide range of ages. Many of these games can teach children to read better, and parents know precisely how vital reading is to children and the future of their children.

Games are great ways to help children into reading, even if they do not like to read. They engage your children and apply a different method of teaching. It is a great way to find out how your child learns as every child thrives in different learning styles. Children often find games exciting and fun, but they have no idea that you may also be helping them build their reading skills. Different games on the market can help children build their reading vocabulary, but the most important thing to remember is to make playing whatever type of game fun for children.

Animal Flash Cards are great for teaching young children to read. These flashcards have incredible pictures of animals, and on each card is an animal. These flashcards allow parents to ask their children to tell them what animal it is and depending on the child's age, they can ask the child to say the letter the name of the animal begins with or have the child spell the name of the animal. There are many flashcards on the market for children of all ages, such as alphabet flashcards, number flashcards, and even simple math flashcards.

Teaching your children their ABC's can be easy and a lot of fun for the children as well as the parents. There are a variety of games that will help children to learn their ABC's by featuring uppercase letters with their appropriate lowercase letter printed on special flash cards. There are even building blocks with the uppercase letter and the lowercase letter that can help children learn how to read and spell while having a blast building and creating with those building blocks.

Basic board games should not be written off as a waste of time like many adults tend to do. They serve as a great way to teach children to have fun while they are learning. There is a large variety of board games available on the market today that include Trouble, Sorry, Memory, Monopoly, Life, and so many more. Each of these games and every game on the market has the age limit for children, which will help parents know what games are more appropriate for their children, as children get older it is important to continue introducing new board games to them, which will enable them to continue building their reading vocabulary.

Game markers are designing games today so that they integrate playing while learning, and the good thing is that game makers have figured out how to kill two birds with one stone without letting the children realize that they are learning. When children play the available games on the market, parents learn that the games teach their children brand new skills. Helping children to develop skills is a good idea to mix with having fun while spending time with their family playing these games.

There are a lot of interactive games for children that you can utilize for their development and learning. Playing games that incorporate school subjects or develop their analytical and problem-solving skills is a great way to strengthen a range of skill sets and boost self-esteem. Here are a few of the top reasons to use interactive educational games for children:

1. Games are objective or goal-driven, so kids will develop an understanding that to succeed, they

must meet or exceed the goal by following objectives.

2. Games introduce subject matter in a fun, pressure-free way, which makes it less intimidating. Learning in a structured environment can sometimes be intimidating and open up a world of insecurities and worry for kids.
3. Interactive games encourage problem-solving. No matter the subject, learning games provide ample opportunity for children to practice problem-solving. They'll learn about trial-and-error, how to show their work, and experiment until they've found the right answer.
4. Games also develop critical thinking and analytics, especially when the strategy is involved. Kids will learn how to evaluate what they did, learn from their mistakes, and try again. It encourages children to take in success and failures and learn to strive to do better next time.
5. Children learn social skills as they play games with others. They learn to build relationships and trust the importance of teamwork and cooperation. As much as parents and adults are vital to a child's development, spending time with children within a similar age gap helps kids learn to socialize.
6. Interacting with others helps them understand how

others feel and how to deal with emotions. New social situations are crucial for a child's development as it exposes them to the diversity of the world and gives them experience in learning social cues.

7. Children also learn about competition, winning, and losing gracefully. The most important lesson that kids can learn is how to accept defeat but persevered the next time to try again until they are successful and meet their goals.

8. Games have instructions and guidelines, so children get practice reading and listening to certain parameters or restrictions that they need to pay attention to.

9. Games require strategy, which makes the players more active participants. This means when kids are playing academically interactive games, and they are more engaged than when they simply are doing worksheets. Thinking strategically is a great way to practice critical thinking and problem solving, which are skills that kids will take well into adulthood.

10. Playing interactive games for children is a wonderful way to spend quality time with your kids. And as adults, you can learn a lot too!

Games and childhood always go together. Kids use creative games and play to learn and acquire new skills. Creative learning games help them to handle difficult situations and to have lots of fun at the same time. Most kids will create their games, and every new idea is always welcome. Every child is born with creative potential. It is the parents' responsibility to nurture their children with the right original games to improve a child's creativity and the ability to interact. Although parents must be responsible for the safety of a child during playtime while allowing some leeway for learning to occur, it isn't easy to try to balance. This will allow the child to be more imaginative, and it will help them learn to do things on their own.

Fostering creativity is often placed at the backburner of a child's development, whether intentionally or not. Some parents don't see the value in creative skills, while some simply forget about it. However, understand that nurturing creativity within your child is crucial and branches out into almost every aspect of their lives. Additionally, creative thinking will follow them into their adult lives when they enter the workforce and beyond. Creative thinking has a slew of benefits. By fostering any creative talents, kids can abstractly, fluidly practice thinking outside of the box. It also places an importance on originality and encourages your children to let loose and think freely. Between structured schooling and extracurricular activities, having the downtime to explore their surroundings in an imaginative way which significantly helps reduce overworking kids and promotes brain health.

Creative and dramatic play is one of the bestways for kids to express themselves. They are free to express the way they feel inside. Every day, children tend to imitate animals, machines, and older people. It helps them understand and work within their environment. Parents can encourage their children with toys and games. They should choose the right types of toys and games for their age range. Examples of simple yet creative games for kids include reading a story and acting it out afterward. This helps to enhance a child's ability to imagine and portray basic roles in life.

Most creative learning games for kids' games require physical energy and movements. Most of these games should be played outdoors. Parents should always remember that playing should always be fun and memorable. If the usual games you play with your kids seem boring and tiresome, then why not try the games listed above and let your creativity take over. These creative games for kids will surely make every child's day fun and enjoyable.

Every human, especially a child, enjoys playing and have fun. It is one great way for a kid to interact with other kids. Playing is a source of relaxation while simultaneously being the stimulation of one's brain and body. Playing creative games for kids is a sure way to develop a child's creativity, imagination, problem-solving skills, and mental growth and awareness.

Learning games for children is a great way to capture your child's attention while practicing a learned skill. Whether you are using a game to introduce a new subject to your child or going over a subject they've learned about in school for familiarity, there are plenty of ways learning games for children can benefit your child in addition to the academics.

Games also do not have to break the bank, as many parents fear. They can be simple exercises that require no tools or props at all or can go the opposite way and be as elaborate as you might like. For many parents, simply leaving their kids to their own devices to come up with their own play is the best way for them to practice thinking outside the box and often yields the best and most entertaining results for your kids.

Problem-solving: No matter the subject, learning games provide ample opportunity for children to practice problem-solving. They'll learn about trial-and-error, how to show their work, and experiment until they've found the right answer. Learning games for children are also a good avenue for children to learn how to evaluate what they did, learn from their mistakes, and try again.

Social Skills: Children learn social skills as they work with other kids. They learn to build relationships and trust. They get to learn the importance of teamwork and cooperation in achieving a particular goal or objective embedded with the game. Interacting with others helps them understand how others feel and how to deal with emotions. Children also learn about competition, winning, and losing gracefully. The most important lesson that kids can learn is how to accept defeat but still try again.

Comprehension Skills: Games have instructions and guidelines, so children get to practice reading and listening to certain parameters or restrictions that they need to pay attention to.

Learning games for children are a great way to learn more about academic subjects, develop important skills, and have fun! The natural enjoyment of playing a game is heightened by the benefits of encouraging your child's natural curiosity. Educational games are especially beneficial for teaching your kids in a pressure-free environment. While school may develop an internalized anxiety as they face the pressure of their peers and teachers observing them, games instead completely take away this factor but have the benefit of your child practising these skills that are important for them to succeed.

Parents have found that math games, in particular, have been incredibly helpful for their young children. Many parents face the issue of their children having difficulty adapting to mathematics in school and struggling to understand concepts. For one parent, she found that her young son was particularly struggling with his multiplication tables. He had been doing poorly in his tests despite her scolding him and taking away his electronics to get him to memorize them. Despite the drills and activity sheets, he was too discouraged and had developed anxiety from the pressure which turned into a fear for the maths that only grew as time went on and he continued to do poorly. The mother decided to switch her tactics. Instead of continually berating him and criticizing him for not doing well, she ended taking a different approach by trying to turn learning into a fun thing. She ended up finding some math resource websites on the Internet that had plenty of multiplication games. They used his failed quizzes as a starting point to identify his weaknesses and where his consistent mistakes were. Her son was already enticed from the fact that he was being encouraged to play games on the computer.

Additionally, she took to playing multiplication games with him, forgoing his textbook altogether. After some time of consistent practice and positive reinforcement, her son ended up getting a far better grasp on the concept and did well on his evaluations. The key here was that she took a proactive approach to her son's learning and really sat down and took the time to work with him, rather than continually scolding him for his failures.

Educational flash games are activities made for children from three to twelve years old. These are very simple games with simple mechanics that entertain and educate your child simultaneously. These activities feature interactive and colorful characters, animals, shapes, and objects to get the attention of learning children. Unlike the common flash entertainment found online, which has mature content, educational flash entertainment has interesting and educational themes that children would love.

Requirements to Play

Any decent computer or notebook with at least 1.0 GHz of processing power and 512mb of ram could play these games hassle-free. These games use the internet browser as their platform and run using the Adobe Flash engine for their graphics and audio. If you don't have access to a computer, consider visiting the library as they generally have some computer setups geared towards children.

Where to find Educational Flash Games

Prongo is a very popular website that provides quality and educational flash games for children. They have specific flash games for different age brackets. These games may start from basic color recognition and mouse training to more challenging games like memory and math games. Prongo provides educational games for children of different ages.

Here are two of the best educational games for Ages 3 to 6 years old:

Colorful Shape Making Game - Activities let your children stamp their shapes. Kids learn basic shapes while creating their pieces of art. This game is perfect for children learning to use the mouse, learning basic shapes, and those who want to be creative.

8-Planets, The Solar System Game – Activities let your child create their solar system. It's suitable for children learning the names of the solarsystem. The game features colorful interactive planets that make learning about the solar system fun for hours.

Here are two of the best educational games for Ages 6 to nine years old:

Copycat Jack Game - This is a memory type game that can provide many hours of fun for your little one. The child must recall the colors in the order that it was shown in the game. Activities include colorful animation and animal sounds to reinforce the child's memory.

Batter's Up Baseball - This is a mathematics type game to help improve your child's math skills. The game will show a simple math problem that your little one must solve. Your child must click the right answer within the time limit. This flash game is suitable for children learning basic multiplication and division.

Here is an educational game for Ages 9 to 12 years old:

Farm Stand - This website is excellent for practising multiplication and addition skills. The site has fundamental yet challenging math problems for pre-teens.

But there are plenty of games on the Internet that are also continually evolving and becoming more intuitive as technology continues to advance. Children now have access to tablets and smartphones, which have hundreds of educational apps to teach them new skills in a fun and engaging way. As a parent, be sure to monitor these apps before giving them to your children to make sure all the content is appropriate and at a suitable level for your child. Many parents choose to rely on lists curated explicitly by teachers to find apps that would be best suited for their child in whichever age range they might be. Additionally, this is a perfect time to educate your children on the Internet and some of the dangers that lie in sharing private information. Ensure that parental locks are in place and be sure to restrict access to inappropriate websites.

Letting your children play educational flash games is a very efficient and enjoyable way of learning. With full player interaction, colorful objects, and interesting audio effects, the child would not be bored and would be very interested in playing the games.Letting them learn is key to their success.

Teaching children to spell is often not an easy task. For teachers and parents, it is a difficult challenge. Today's means of helping pupils learn more words involves using multiple teaching strategies to make learning more meaningful to children. Spelling is one of the important aspects of learning English words. It is integral in language development because the aptitude in spelling determines much of the individual's writing abilities. It must be taken into account that language skills can fall as writing and speaking abilities, and these are separate entities. Someone may speak fluently but commit misspellings. Hence, in the total development of one's linguistic faculties, spelling training is an important discipline.

Kids being taught of words can display signs of boredom or difficulty, but learning how to spell does not have to be tough, as there are lots of fun ways for kids to learn words and become familiar with their spellings. The most effective way for children to spell words correctly is to have frequent, meaningful experiences. This can be achieved by using the words in writing compositions. The more frequently a child gets to see the words, the more they become familiar with its spelling.

Nevertheless, learning spelling can also become more fun using games that kids will enjoy doing. Word games like Boggle and Scrabble help kids get a good grasp with different words, as they form words using tiles for Scrabble and identifying word formations in Boggle. This can sharpen their spelling and word formation and identification skills, which becomes useful in practical applications, not just inside English classes. Parents can help their children during wordsearch games so that they don't feel like they have to do the game alone. After all, if a game feels like it tires them mentally, they may find it frustrating. The best way to stimulate their mind is to give them a challenge. But you can be their aid by providing hints and clues.

Spelling bees can be your family's fun routine, and this can involve everyone in the family to help the child develop good learning habits even at home. You can give each other words to spell and give the child simple words to spell out orally. Of course, allow him or her to give you words to spell, too. This does not have to appear as though it were planned. You can do spelling bees while sitting in the living room or enjoying a car ride. In other words, fill in vacant or even dreary moments with spelling bees, which the child can enjoy. These activites, while some may regard as pointless, give your children ample opportunity to practice their skills in a non-pressured environment.

If you have a computer at home ,you can download spelling game software. Interactive online spelling games for children allows convenient usage of educational games at domestic confines. You can turn the computer on and leave the child to play on their own or play with them for some fun bonding. Another advantage of educational computer games is that you don't need any other material but the PC. Word hunt, Bookworm, Food Jumble, Word Mojo, and Text Twist are some of the games that can be downloaded to your PC and played by your children during vacant hours. Each of these games comes with instructions that you should explain to your child. Make sure they know how to play the game before actually allowing them to play. If the child plays without grasping the instructions, they would be lost, and the sole purpose of the game is just forfeited.

Games are just some of the tools to help children learn better. Besides learning to spell, they should be able to use the words in conversations and writing compositions. Application of what they have learned is an effective way of locking in the learned words in their memory.

If you are interested in purchasing outdoor family games for children, you will be pleased to know that there are many benefits associated with these activities. In today's world of rapidly evolving levels of technology and virtual opportunities, outdoor play, and entertainment is being placed on the low end of different types of entertainment opportunities for families. It is important to understand that traditional family outdoor games provide a wide array of opportunities for children, such as developing certain skills, physical fitness, and developmental milestones. In this book, you will learn the different benefits associated with outdoor family games for children.

Physical Development and Maintenance

One of the most important aspects of a child's life is their physical growth and development. It has been established that children who play various types of games in an outdoor environment are more likely to have higher levels of strength and optimal stamina than children who do not spend a lot of time playing outdoors. The muscles of the body become stronger, and the tissues can heal themselves more quickly in physically active children. In addition to this, the organs and other aspects of the body are properly maintained. They can get the oxygen and nutrients that they require when a child engages in outdoor physical activities. Furthermore, it is important to understand that outdoor family games can strengthen the child's immune system and keep their health in check.

Mental Development

Family outdoor games often require a person to follow certain rules and regulations. In addition to this, the games often require the child to place their focus on a certain goal to completion. These games provide a wonderful opportunity for a child to grow mentally. Not only do outdoor games increase the amount of oxygen that is getting to the brain so that it may stay healthy, but children are also learning how to follow procedures, are required to stay organized, and are improving their concentration efforts. Additionally, fun family outdoor games provide a child with the opportunity to increase their creativity levels and better understand the world around them.

Social Development

Family games that are played outdoors provide children with the opportunity to interact socially with their family members and perhaps even other people that they are friends with or live near to. Children will learn how to take turns with other individuals and share in a common interest. They will also gain an understanding of the importance of rules and guidelines. Many children will benefit from the fact that they will have to communicate with others while playing games in an outdoor environment. Games provide children with the opportunity to achieve quick success. In turn, this success will allow them to experience a higher level of confidence within themselves.

Many parents have found that getting involved with their own kids outdoors has had significant effects on their own mental and physical health in addition to their children's, which is also just as important. As much as you want your child to interact with their own cohort and gather more experiences outside of the household bubble, spending time with your children fosters a strong bond and encourages them to communicate with you. Families are crucial to a child's development as they provide a consistent source of care and love, and they associate safety with their own family. So being a constant that encourages the strengthening of this relationship is so essential as your kid's age and go through the various stages of life and experience all of the changes around them. It can be incredibly overwhelming, so spending time with them not only for their own education but also for their mental health is vital. For parents, as important as it is to take care of your children, don't forget to take care of yourselves either. Your mental well-being should also be a priority, so always factor that in as you factor in your child's.

HEART HEALTHY ACTIVITIES FOR KIDS

Today, more and more children are overweight, and many suffer from obesity. The numbers are staggering and incredibly worrying for parents raising young, impressionable children. In a world where fast food is becoming increasingly accessible, and our adherence to technology is making us more stagnant, heart health is becoming a growing issue among the youth. There have been so many technological advancements that have made life much simpler today, but this has made life more comfortable and has contributed to laziness among many young people today. Many children today are not understanding the importance of exercising enough and are in poor health. Some claim that children must be more involved. You may be looking for safe cardiac activities for children. You can do many things to help your children get the exercise they need.

Go Out More

Today, children are inside more than ever. With television, video games, computers, and a host of music players, children do not feel the need to come out and have fun. You should allow your children to go out. When outside, they can run, cycle, climb and do all kinds of safe cardiac exercises. Let your children get dirty outside. Parents have a fear for germs and diseases in the outside world, choosing instead to shelter their children indoors and keep them dormant. But germs are a natural product of the world. While we have to educate our children to be mindful and wash their hands and practice safe sanitization, preventing them from exploring the outside environment is just as important.

You should schedule trips with your family for walks or campsites. During physical activity, children can exercise and burn calories and strengthen their muscles. Getting involved along with your kids gives them an example to look up to.

Get Involved in Sports

Sports are a perfect place for children to train and put their bodies to use. Plus, kids find playing sports fun, so they'll enjoy the workout. It will take your children some time to find a sport that they want to commit to. But with so many sports available to choose from, your child is bound to find something they will enjoy. As not all sports activities are for all kids, taking the time to find a sport that they will enjoy and appreciate will yield better results.

Of course, children may be interested in sports for the wrong reason. You should tell them that sport is about having fun and practising teamwork while exercising and that it is not just about winning. Sports activities can be beneficial in many ways for youngsters.

Possibly your children will engage in a host of sporting in your area. Leagues for your children will be supported by recreational centers, schools, and other organizations. Some Leagues can be more competitive than others, so you can see which league suits well.

Be Creative

Be innovative as you know your children best. You can find many safe activities for children and do not be afraid to use the resources available to you, such as the Internet to find free ideas and inspiration on good ways to get your kids active. Your children may not always be inspired to be healthy, but they can be encouraged to develop healthier behaviours that will be more sustainable for years to come. Many children resist their parent's attempts to get them to be more active, but this is where you have to persist. While your children may not be grateful to you right now, ageing brings along more wisdom and they will eventually be more understanding at your attempts to live a healthy lifestyle.

Ways to keep your child's heart-healthy

Take responsibility for your child's heart health by cultivating behaviours that profit later in life. According to Colin Kane, M.D., Children's health, and Director of Cardiology Outreach at UT Southwestern, the most successful way to do this is by making healthy living a priority for the entire family.

"If the child sees that it is vital to his mother, dad, and other family members to eat well and to have enough exercise, he/she will be more likely to follow the same lifestyle." "Telling the child to eat carrots and celery is not reasonable when they see other relatives eating French fries. Likewise, if the child sees mom and dad watching lots of televisions, they would probably do the same thing.

How to raise a heart-healthy child

- Keep moving: exercise as a family, cycling, walking, swimming, or playing outdoor sports. If you're cooped up inside all day, take breaks often to stretch and move around.
- Complimentary: Enjoy your heart's wellbeing with

your family events or stroll to a park to have a healthy picnic. Keep successes to cultivate a healthy sense of self-esteem.

- Limit time: Excess screening leads to a sedentary lifestyle and continuous snacks that raise the risk of obesity and cardiovascular illness. Limit the number of hours a day for Cable, computer, and telephone.
- Schedule pre-sport checks: If your child is an athlete, please visit your child's paediatrician for a physical examination to rule out sudden heart death. Although this is rare in generally stable teens; otherwise, it must be discussed to recognize those at risk.
- Go to the grocery store together: learn more about the foods that contribute to your children growing stronger and make it fun for them. Staples of wheat or whole grains, low-fat dairy products, meat, fish, and nuts should be 100% in your kitchen.
- Keep on hand nutritious choices: Give your child healthy snacks, including whole-grain crackers and string cheese, hummus dip and vegetables, Greek yoghurt with apple slices, nuts, and dried fruit, whenever they come home from school.
- Make dinner a family affair: get your child interested in preparing and planning meals. The

kitchen can be an excellent school for your kids as it teaches them discipline but gets them involved with cooking and baking. It's a great way to teach them some independence while getting them excited to eat healthily.
- Check for salt: Avoid processed foods and keep saltshakers away from the table. A lot of foods and seasonings have added sodium in them, so be wary of this.
- Keep involved: be your child's advocate and others. Insist on safe school food options. Ensure that your child's paediatrician controls cardiovascular factors such as BMI, blood pressure, and cholesterol. Message elected authorities on heart problems. Make your voice heard.
- Set realistic targets and constraints. Small steps and incremental improvements can make a massive difference over time in your child's health.

For many, parenting has been entirely a learning process. Recognize that there is nothing wrong with that. Some parents have struggled to strike a balance of healthy eating in their household while adhering to budget constraints as eating organic and fresh ingredients is not as realistic for many. As parents have grown alongside their kids, they have learnt the adverse effects junk food and processed foods will have on their children in the long run and have been taking steps to slowly remove these foods as staples in their diet, replacing them with vegetables and fruits instead. The gradual process takes some time, as children quickly adapt to the foods that they enjoy and often latch onto them, especially if they are sodium and MSG-filled. However, some parents have implemented more greens into their kids' diets by taking the time to make homecooked meals. Many parents, especially those on a budget, choose to meal prep as it is more cost and time-efficient for busy working parents and have reached a point to limit fast food to once a month.

MIND-BLOWING EXERCISE GAMES TO MAKE KIDS ACTIVE, FIT & HEALTHY

Parents, I'm sure you're going to agree fitness exercises can be perfect for children because they can help them remain healthy and fit in the long term. These days, children live more of a sedentary lifestyle with the changing trends. The type of lifestyle they currently lead will lead to diverse health issues for them as they get older.

We have had a more 'involved' childhood than today's digital generation.

As a mom, I'm sure that you have found yourself wondering at some point if your kid is getting enough workout or not.

But don't worry! Don't worry! We'll help you with ingenious exercise game ideas to try at home!

MIND-BLOWING EXERCISE GAMES TO MAKE KIDS ... | 277

It is an immense challenge to keep kids off digital devices with screens' introduction – let alone taking them out and play actively.

And with so many interactive games and events, we can't blame them, can we? TV and video games are made to entice your children and keep them hooked for hours on end. It's a constant battle for parents between the electronic devices and getting them outside for fresh air and exercise.

And now what? Ban your child's digital devices? Ah, we're pretty sure that will backfire. All this increases your child's rebellious behaviour.

We can't encourage our kids to grow unsafe and unhealthy at the same time!

What we should do is make physical exercise more fun. Make physical activity as exciting as a video game with the added benefit of the training, releasing endorphins into your child's brains. This hormone makes them feel happy and healthy.

We need to avoid health issues such as our child being underweight. The only choice we had in our days was to play these exercise games with our mates. Not only are they good for your physical health but also your mental well-being.

It teaches kids to be more social, be a team player, and instil valuable leadership skills. These skills will follow them into their adult life and is crucial for their successful development.

Let's look at some fun activities and games that your child can easily take part in to improve their physical health.

We have ideas for both indoor and outdoor exercise games, so take a look!

EXERCISE ACTIVITIES TO GET YOUR CHILD FIT & HEALTHY:: RACES:

You can arrange races with a small reward for your child and their friends in a yard or field around your home. These are a great way to involve your child and all of their friends because the concept is simple enough for children to grasp an1d easy for the adults to plan and prepare for.

Be imaginative with the game. You have a three-legged, one-legged, crab-walking race, and so on. Also, let's not forget the classic race of settling on a finish point that's a little far off, and every path can be used to get there and see who wins. Jump rope (skipping rope) races are fantastic, too, as its full leg exercise combined with a cardio workout.

The possibilities here are endless. Spending time outside can be as elaborate or as simple as you and your children want. Be sure to get involved yourself. Seeing their parents take part in activities really encourages children to change a negative mindset and motivates them to want to participate.

Sports:

Almost always, your child is naturally drawn to a sport. You can see by what they are watching and what sport video games they may be playing.

Have a game with them mostly for this specific sport. Enrol and invite the kids to join their school team. Some activities, such as swimming, should undoubtedly encourage your child to exercise regularly.

Swimming is a great activity and is extremely versatile as it can be done solo or with a group of friends. Make a sunny summer fun day, and your kids will undoubtedly be excited. If it is winter, you can even find an indoor pool at a leisure center.

Scavenger Hunt

It can be indoors or outdoors, but scavenger hunts are a great way to entice your children into exploring their environments, and of course, being more active.

Organize a hunt that extends over an extensive area or even inside your house.

Just place the toys or treats concealed in various places and start your child first.

There should be a puzzle written for each location. If you make sure that the places are far apart, your kids will run around.

GARDENING:

Free practices such as gardening are a great source of kids' exercise. This does not mean you need to own a greenhouse by any means. Simply take some pots, some saplings, and some mud and ask your kids to fill their jars and teach them about regular watering and caring for your plants. Educate them on the basic sciences that are involved when caring for plants outside.

Dance:

Dance is the simplest and one of the most exciting activities to cover your daily cardio exercise. Dance is an incredible way to get your kids moving, whether it's through structured lessons or merely putting on their favourite music and letting loose. It can improve the condition of the heart, lungs, and overall endurance. It promotes better coordination and flexibility while improving musicality. It's a simple way to encourage movement and does not require much preparation or tools.

Walking:

If you have a dog, share the everyday activities of walking. It promotes consistent activity every day and is a great way to get regular fresh air.

Hula Hooping:

Children love hula hoops. They are inexpensive to purchase and are great for all ages. For new learners, they're a challenging enough activity that will really engage them. For seasoned hula hoopers, they are a great exercise to get your heart rate up.

Get some hula hoops for your kids and start hooping with them.

Blow off that steam.

We're used to our kid's throwing tantrums. What if I told you something would support them both mentally and physically when they are in a good mood?

It may sound very out of the box, but when they kick and jump and whine, they get tired because of their energy.

It also lets them get all their rage and frustration out without even noticing it.

EXERCISE GAMES FOR KIDS THAT ARE ABSOLUTE FUN:

Follow the leader:

When you play this game, you will be the leader, and it is the best way for your kids to do a good workout. Ensure that exercises such as jumping jacks, kicks, running, and jumps are included.

Tag:

A simple tag game where you chase your kids and, if you catch anyone, you have to chase them, is a fun way to train old schools. There are dozens of variants of tag, like "Freeze" and "Cops and Robbers". Considering spicing up these classic games with your own new rules.

Capture the Flag:

"Capture the Flag" is a classic game that will surely keep your kids entertained and involved for a long time. Gather the friends of your child and bring them to a large area with plenty of closed spaces to hide. Divide them into two teams and give each group a flag to cover what the other team wants to find.

Hopscotch:

Hopscotch is a fun game they can play either indoor (using tiles assigned) and outdoor (with chalk on a sidewalk or pavement). Continue to make the hopscotch course bigger and bigger to keep your kids involved and excited about jumping.

Twister:

There are varieties of the twister mat game in different toy shops and online stores. It's the ideal kids' indoor fitness game, so it's a smart idea to invest in it, and it won't break the bank. Kids of all ages enjoy this game.

Table Tennis:

It is good to opt into a table tennis table for another great opportunity for indoor exercise.

Any tiny, mostly vacant room can be used for table tennis, and since it requires a lot of running, it's a great way to practice. You can even find a smaller table with your child and friends if your child is very young.

POP, POP.

Inspired by some simple birthday matches, you have to blow some bubbles out in your garden and ask your child to pop them all.

Another major factor of the game is that the balloon does not hit the ground (which, of course, does not last for more than a second).

QUICK TIPS:

There are a variety of things you need to consider while taking kids to practice because it's not the most straightforward task.

Schedule it right:

Take care to choose a specific time of the day suitable for all moods and free time. Typically, it works best right before or right after lunch. Having a dedicated time for these activities keeps children more motivated and consistent.

Track, chart, and reward progress:

Follow up on all workouts, report the kids' workout-related accomplishments, and earn a little monthly award for the best-performing kid or family member. These are great methods to reinforce these good habits positively.

Enrol in exercise-related events:

If it's a marathon or a boot camp to work out, get your child into it! Events such as these bring more excitement and variety to the workout. Additionally, these are great environments to make friends and find buddies for their activities outside of these places if your child needs a friend with a like-minded hobby.

Even events like a safety training course or a self-defence class promote exercise and build vital skills.

Get your kid involved in planning:

If there is one thing that kids enjoy the most, it's getting involved. Parents often navigate under the impression that they must do everything by themselves, but this certainly doesn't have to be the case. Instead, get your child to be involved in planning out their times to instil organization and responsibility. It will help their imagination flourish by designing something that others will pursue.

Get them to schedule preparation and perhaps even set goals for a week. Give them the reins and autonomy to make decisions within a specific capacity.

Spend more time in open nature:

Whether it's a picnic or just a walk through the park, it's always lovely to spend time in the open. Nature is a free playground, and its beauty is unparalleled, yet people tend to take this for granted. Parents often cite planned activities as being too expensive or too much of a commitment. However, nature is the exact opposite of all of this as there is so much to marvel at in the environment around us. Plan a picnic once every few weeks and take a ball, a frisbee, and a jump rope to keep your kid happy and well trained, if possible.

Exercise for children is beneficial to their welfare. Exercise helps young people absorb their seemingly infinite resources. My kid didn't like the thought of spending time amid the squamous bugs, grass, and lawnmower noises in the first place. How can you get your child off the couch?

Create a positive experience. Do not ask your child to spend 15 to 30 minutes on a child's treadmill or elliptical trainer three days a week. As ridiculous as it sounds, it is not unheard of. It's a sure way to foster resentment in your child and nurture unhealthy patterns of thinking towards for their body image. If your child considers exercise as exercise, they probably won't enjoy it.

Take a "workout" box and pack it into something called a "run"–walking, jumping, gymnastics, dancing, pool, play soccer, and so on–rather than trapped in passive entertainment. You may like the power to walk, but your 8-year-old may hate the idea. Spend energy and involve other children from the neighbourhood with an exciting duck, duck, goose game.

Other fantastic activities for children is to play kickball, whiffle ball, play in the playground, or climb trees. Consider investing in a bicycle or roller-skates for your kids if they show a keen interest in them. These are great ways to get your kids moving.

If your child spends most of his/her time in front of a screen, the outside can look like foreign turf. He/she must emulate your positive and inspiring approach to outdoor activities. So be optimistic and for a while, switching off from the online world. Children's exercise doesn't have to be elaborate; it should just be pleasant.

Moreover, there is no need to give your child a strict workout schedule. Concentrate on having fun with them. Let him/her rest or stop altogether if he/she gets tired after 15 minutes. A moderate dose of 15-minute exercise for both of you will go a long way.

If these guidelines are properly followed, your kids will undoubtedly enjoy physical activity soon enough. The primary factor is to make these activities as enjoyable as possible. These exercise games will automatically attract your kids, and they will soon be enthusiastic about them.

Make sure you are also excited if you want your kids to be. If you're doing a workout at home or outdoors, it can still be an enjoyable way to spend time with your kids or even encourage your kids to socialize with their own friends.

It also helps to explain to your kids the importance of physical exercise at a young age. Understanding why it's essential to them makes your job easier as the parent. Parents often take their child's intelligence for granted and choose to label things as another thing they "must do simply". It's another sure way to get them disinterested and unmotivated because they simply do not see the same benefits as you see. So, remember to educate your children to understand why you continue to push them to do these things. This creates a good foundation for them to eventually take the initiative on their own to get moving, pursue sports and spend time outside. As much as they are at the age where they are encouraged by you, children go through stages of maturity and significant changes, which means that sometimes, your own encouragements will fall to deaf ears. Therefore, establishing a good foundation from a young age to understand health in simple terms and being able to discern between good and bad habits can eventually develop into more fantastic practices well-past childhood.

HEALTHY LIVING LESSONS TO TEACH YOUR KIDS

There are also ways for children to learn how to make safe lifestyle decisions. You can also help them because children look for guidance from their parents and mentors. And in many areas of their wellbeing, it is necessary to enable them to succeed.

While it can seem like an extremely intimidating subject to broach with your children, it certainly does not have to be complicated or overwhelming to teach your children to make healthier choices. As long as you are well-informed and have done your own research, you should be prepared to face all of their questions that arise. Recall that you yourself were a child once and consider what you might have questions about as well. Everything you need to keep your children on track is quick and easy to handle. Working as a family to make good choices is also a great way to improve children's healthy living values.

If you need ideas to bring healthy living principles into practice for children, aim to concentrate on these five high-impact areas:

- Eating a fiber-rich diet
- Enjoying kid-friendly exercises
- Getting adequate sleep
- Keeping good mental health in mind
- Developing a safe, responsible relationship with electronic devices

They absorb new knowledge and learn quickly. Below you can find tips to help children make wise health choices. Before you know it, your children will be able to select healthier choices themselves.

Find Ways to Help Your Kids Eat More Fiber

Children need healthy meals and snacks to promote their play and development. The secret to renewable energy for fueling days of fun is fiber-rich food. The value of fiber is already understood to adults. When you are grown-up, you've heard "eat more fiber " too much to count. Take your wisdom and teach your children why they need it, also.

It begins with a simple fact: without fiber, it is much harder to digest the food you consume correctly. To help health digestion, a child (as in any adult) requires sufficient fluids and fiber. If the digestive system runs low, constipation and pain could be on the horizon. And it's challenging to run and play with pain in your stomach.

It's not enough to help save digestion. After a meal, children are happy with fiber-packed food. It encourages fullness and helps to discourage children from overeating. With fiber, your children receive regular quantities of energy without crashing high sugar levels. Doing this allows children to play or learn more with constant energy.

Help your children see how much fiber per day they need. The recommended daily amounts of fiber for each age group are different. Age plus five grams are the best way to measure the daily fiber required. So, this means that a young person of three needs eight grams of dietary fiber per day.

Fiber is an essential part of many tasty foods and treats that children enjoy. Nuts are excellent fiber sources. All children's friendly fiber foods include; strawberries, beans, bananas, pears, peas, and whole grain. Foods with plenty of fiber provide an extra benefit. Since fiber is naturally found in fruits and vegetables, vitamins and nutrients loaded into fiber-rich foods. Take the time to demonstrate to your children why fiber is necessary and how good it tastes.

You can also slip extra fibers into the baked good or treat them occasionally. Do this by substituting white flour for whole wheat or adding more fruits and vegetables to sauces and other dishes. Such modifications can go a long way to satisfy the fiber needs of your child.

One excellent way to help children consume the fiber they need is to provide five suitable portions of fruit and veggies per day. Portions generally coincide with what age group your child falls in. Be mindful of the fact that the older they get, the larger and denser the foods become. If children eat their fruits and veggies and other fiber -rich foods every day, there is no need to count fiber grams.

Make Exercise Fun for Your Kids (and for You)

Children are now moving and grooving experts. They run, jump, climb, and play all day long — this is an expected next step for children to go about as soon as they can walk.

An exercise that appears to play is a perfect way to inspire children to be involved. And it doesn't take a ride to the gym for children to travel. Instead, it would help if you went to the park or playground.

The best child-friendly exercises are flexibility, power, and stamina.

Tag and foot racing games are ideal for teaching children agility and speed. Sports such as football, basketball, and running help children concentrate on stamina. Tumbling improve versatility.

Children will flex their strength on monkey bars or jungle fitness centers. Jumping hoops, driving on a teeter-totter, and pushing friends on the swing set are other enjoyable things to create power.

But don't allow their ability to play prevent you from keeping them safe. Children can get injured just like adults do as they play. That is why children need to be taught how to protect their tiny muscles and joints from injury.

Encourage your children to warm up before a match. Warming up activities may include a stroll to the park or a short series of yoga. Stop dehydration by ensuring plenty of water. Check regularly with children so that no symptoms of injuries are missed.

One of the best things you can do is let your children practice. Show them how critical healthy activity is—making workouts a family business can also encourage children to build a sustainable interest in health and fitness. It also encourages children to explore new ways of travelling. Go out and play together and enjoy the family workout.

For many parents, they have learned that exercise does not have to be as dreaded as it usually is. By involving their children in a daily routine, it isn't treated as a chore. Instead, it merely becomes an integral part of their day. Instead of constantly reminding their children to exercise, parents simply enforce activities like taking a stroll around their neighbourhood as part of their norm. Encouraging your kids to move does not have to be like pulling teeth. It can be as mindless and obvious as breakfast. It simply becomes a part of everyone's day. As fun as planning activities and organizing events can be, treating it as another opportunity to spend time with your family can take away the negative connotation that often accompanies the notion of "exercise". Everyone's journey with their bodies is entirely different. Fostering a good relationship between body, mind, and soul for your children starts with you. Be a good role model to them and emulate a mindset that is healthy and positive so that your children learn how to cope well with their continually changing bodies.

Particularly within the youth, eating disorders and a myriad of body image issues come hand in hand with growing up and puberty. As a parent, being empathetic and sensitive to their struggles is hugely crucial. Sometimes kids don't want to be told what to do. Instead, they need someone to rely on to navigate through the mental turmoil they may be facing. The key here is to prioritize mental health as much as you give physical health importance because the two go hand in hand with each other and can affect each other significantly.

Being able to have a serious talk with your child about body image can significantly benefit them and how they perceive themselves, so be ready to sit down and discuss the notions of "fat" and "thin" and how body shaming negatively affects the mind. Try to reduce the stigma around health and weight by approaching the subject with empathy and respectfully. As your children age, having these serious conversations with them are crucial and you should be prepared to say the right things.

HEALTHY SLEEP HABITS FOR KIDS

A good night's sleep is about dreaming and experiencing all the stages of sleep. Most kids wake up themselves in the morning if they sleep well enough. The importance of sleep is often brushed off because its negative impacts don't appear immediately. But over time, as we age and continue unhealthy practices, we can significantly affect how we age and how our body reacts to maturing.

Sleep is a powerful healing cycle. It improves our physical, emotional, mental, and metabolic health. It helps us combine and unite our memories and has a direct impact on our behaviour. Sleep heals us and allows our bodies to revitalize after a day of being put to the extremes.

So, as expected, a poor sleep habit will lead to reduced efficiency to do well in school. Children who have a poor sleeping habit might even be mistaken for having attention-deficit hyperactivity disorder (ADHD). When kids don't get enough sleep, they have a problem with concentration in class, they get easily distracted, and be more impulsive or hyperactive. As your children age, new external forces are at play that can affect their sleep. Homework, afterschool activities, screen time and an increasingly hectic lifestyle, can contribute to a lack of sleep. For these reasons, we have to ensure that we establish a healthy relationship with sleep early on and stress the absolute importance of consistent and restful sleep.

The Basics of Sleep Hygiene

Sleep is necessary, but for many of us children and adults alike, we simply don't get enough. One of the best ways to get back on track is to improve your sleep habits. In other words, building habits that promote sound sleep quality, such as introducing a routine.

Routines vary depending on the age group. For example, babies are not born with the same body clock that allows us to sleep at night and wake up during the day. In contrast, babies sleep for hours and then wake up for hours anytime. This sleep routine is perfectly normal behaviour for newborns, so parents should keep their natural sleeping routines. To prevent your child from getting overtired, parents should reinforce their natural sleep pattern about an hour after waking up. Parents can also help their child reduce desirable sleep patterns by placing the child in a sunny room during the day and darkroom at night. Eventually, this practice will improve their sleeping habits.

Tips for Healthy Sleeping Habits

Here are tips to improve sleeping habits in children:

Make sufficient sleep a family priority

Endeavour to learn the benefits of getting enough sleep and how a poor sleep routine affects the overall health of your family, especially the kids. Keep in mind that you are to set good examples and guidelines to your children. Habits such as staying up all night with your kids, helping them with their homework is not sending the right message to them.

Starting with you, make sleep a priority for the family. Put away your electronic devices and take time to wind down with your family. Treat bedtime as a sacred time in the household, where everyone follows through with their nightly routines to get to sleep. This way, you teach your children that it's a crucial aspect of a healthy lifestyle – like eating wholesome meals and exercising regularly.

Keep a regular daily routine

A routine that begins every night at the same time supports healthy sleep habits. A bath, story, and bed routine will make young children feel ready to sleep. For older children, a peaceful conversation with you about the day, then relax alone until lights out. Prioritize putting screens away. Keep calm and implement a relaxing mood together before going to bed.

Relax before bedtime

Encourage your child before bedtime to relax. Older kids may want to relax by reading a book, listening to soft music, or breathing. If it takes your child more than 30 minutes to sleep, it will take longer to wind down before the light goes off to sleep. TV, laptops and phones should be put away to allow our brains to rest before we fall asleep. Screens often have the opposite effect by keeping us awake and scrolling for hours on end. Implement a rule to avoid screen time right before bed.

Keep regular sleep and wake times

Hold the bedtime and wake-up times of your child in 1-2 hours per day. Doing this helps keep the body clock in a daily pattern for your infant. For weekends and holidays as well as for school days, this is a smart idea.

Keep older children's naps early and short

Most kids quit napping at the age of 3-5. If you ever eat during the day for more than five years, try to keep the nap no more than 20 minutes and no later than early afternoon. Longer naps can make sleeping difficult for children.

Make sure your child feels safe at night

If your kid is afraid to go to bed or to be in the dark, you should praise your kid and reward them when they are courageous. Avoiding disturbing TV shows, movies, and video games can also support. Some kids who are scared of bedtime feel happier when they have a nightlight, or a door slightly open. Allow your kids to be vulnerable to their fears and take them seriously by trying to find ways to help them manage their anxieties, instead of merely brushing them off. Simply ignoring their fears can have adverse effects on their mental health in the long run.

Check noise and light in your child's bedroom

For good sleep, a quiet, dimly lit room is necessary. Check if the bedroom of your child's sleep is too bright or too noisy. Blue light from TVs, computer screens, phones, and tablets might inhibit melatonin and sleep ability levels. It possibly helps you turn these gadgets off at least one hour before bedtime if you hold your children's screens away at night.

Reduce their workload

Sometimes having a full, hectic schedule can have the opposite effect of tiring out your kids. It can be extremely stressful as they go from one activity to the next and have to do it again tomorrow and the next day. Stress, anxiety and worries can keep children up and keep their brains wide awake as it gets later and later into the night. Consider lessening their workload, especially before bedtime so those evenings can be spent quietly and in preparation for a good night's rest.

Avoid the clock

If the time is frequently checked by your child, ask your child to shift the clock or look out of bed at a place where they cannot see it. Focusing on time and how many minutes have gone by keeps their brain on hyperactive mode. Instead, encourage them to close their eyes and concentrate on some meditative tactics like their breathing to calm down and relax into sleep.

Eat the right amount at the right time

Ensure that your children have a healthy dinner at a decent time if they are feeling hungry or too full before bed; this may be uncomfortable for your child. Doing this can make sleeping difficult for your child. In the morning, you will start your child's body clock at the right time with a nutritious breakfast. Ensuring they are well-fed with healthy food can be crucial to a restful sleep.

Get plenty of natural light in the day

Encourage your kid, especially in the morning, to get as much natural light as possible during the day. Bright light destroys melatonin. This gesture makes your child feel awake and relaxed and tired throughout the day.

Avoid caffeine

In energy drinks, coffee, tea, chocolate, and cola, caffeine is included. Dissuade your child from reaching for these drinks as caffeine itself can have its own effects on young children. However, if they must, encourage your child in the late afternoon and evening to stop those consuming these beverages, as they can completely derail sleep schedules and keep your children up until the wee hours of the night.

Teaching Children How to Make Their Mental Health A Priority

Everyone has emotional ups and downs — even children. As children grow in the big, scary world and experience all of these new sensations and feelings, it can be too overwhelming. That is why it is vital to help children develop a foundation for good mental health in times of anxiety or extreme emotion.

As much as the emphasis is placed on physical health, it is incredibly important to establish equal importance for mental health from the get-go, as this will encourage kids to prioritize both as they age.

It is crucial that you trust what is shared between your relationship with your child. Your child should be able to feel vulnerable with you without fear of being criticized or berated. As a parent or carer, sometimes you have to put aside your feelings to listen without judgement to what your child may be experiencing. Allowing them to get out their entire story and feelings is the first step to successfully managing their emotions, instead of bottling it all up, which can have its own set of disastrous effects.

Children can understand that they have to look after their minds and bodies equally. Feelings of concern, anxiety, depression, and fear all grow up. So, let your children know that they should come to you if they are troubled.

But for your children to trust you as a shoulder to lean on, you must establish a strong bond from their childhood itself. Take time to get to know your children. Parents often overlook this as they are so focused on raising their kids. But parenting is one big balancing act, and being a parent means getting involved in every aspect of your child's life. Have conversations with your child and allow them to be vulnerable without judging them. In that same way, be vulnerable to your own kids and share your own emotions (whether good or bad) with honesty. This does not mean burden them with your problems. But instead, parents should not feel pressure to put on a cheerful façade always. Kids are incredibly wise, and sometimes they can see through your own actions. Instead of trying to combat this, be honest with your kids so that they know to trust you.

Emotional wellness encourages children to feel good about themselves and others. It will allow children to have happier ties. Being honest with your kids tells them that it's okay to be nervous and anxious about new adventures. It's simply a consequence of life. Showing them that you yourself have ups and downs sets them up for realistic expectations as they age. Having well-supported mental wellbeing helps children sleep sufficiently and also excel in their classroom.

It truly all begins with open communication lines. Speak to your children about understanding social and emotional changes. Make sure they know that when they feel negative emotions rising, they can rely on you for guidance. Knowing that someone is continuously supporting them can be extremely encouraging. Furthermore, words of a loved one's affection might be what they need to feel better.

Overall, health is one complicated and interconnected puzzle. By helping your child make wise choices when it comes to their diet and develop healthy habits for exercising, it inadvertently affects their mental health and can make huge improvements. Wholesome foods and daily exercise are the two best ways to keep the mind balanced.

Safe model, Conscientious use of electronic equipment

Digital devices are everywhere, and no doubt, children have easy access to them.

There are two sides to this: either your children use the smartphone or tablet better than you do for relevant activities or waste time with it. What you need to do is guide them through on how to use these devices safely.

Families will ensure that their children are protected online by tracking the usage of mobile phones and tablets and by exchanging passwords. Try to build open contact on the Internet. Please help your child understand what they need to learn, hear, and watch. Say to be careful and never post personal data online.

And managing how long children spend plugged into the digital world is just as critical. Make it a priority to escape screens and machines. These off-screen encounters promote active play and creativity. Implementing such practices helps your family prevent digital pitfalls — such as decreased sleep quality, excessive weight, and weak social skills.

Teach children how to value digital technologies by taking breaks from the technologies themselves. Show kids the value of focusing on the real world around them and be an example of how much you love spending time off your computer by taking the time to talk to them individually.

Find out how to do fun offline things together. There are a myriad of things to do as outlined by this book, but it also exemplifies how important it is to stay away from always being glued to a screen. Exploring the outdoors and different dynamics of your family is a great pairing. Parents often find that their children are more attached to one than the other. Getting active and exploring the outside is a great way to switch up the dynamics and spend one-on-one time with your kids.

Good choices are an effective way for parents to teach their children. Your illustration and advice are adequate to teach you how to make the right decisions. Guide your children to a better life by showing them how to make positive decisions today. Always be aware of the fact that you are your child's example and they are mimicking you, whether intentional or not. Remember this the next time you focus on your cellphone or spend time disengaged from the family. While it places immense pressure on your shoulders, it's an incredible responsibility you have as a parent.

LEAVE A REVIEW!

After reading this book, please feel free to leave a review based on your findings and how useful the guide was to you. I would be incredibly thankful if you could take 60 seconds to write a brief review on Amazon, even if it's just a few sentences!

CONCLUSION

Congratulations! You're a proud parent of lovely little ones. Every day, your child learns and improves his/her physical and mental skills, and you, as a parent, would like to make your best possible efforts to ensure that your child learns from the very start and adopts healthy habits.

After all, it's not that difficult. The main thing to remember is that you do not necessarily transfer genes to your baby as a mom. Your baby learns a lot from you, and if you adhere to a healthy lifestyle, it won't be challenging to help him/her learn. As a responsible parent, it is vital to look after your children's wellbeing and teach them to follow their healthy habits. This practice is the way to avoid infection and to eliminate different diseases.

I hope you've gathered some ideas to instil your child's habits. Following these simple tips, your child can follow a healthy lifestyle from childhood.

Navigating through parenting is a challenging journey that has its own set of euphoric highs and debilitating lows. Parents often struggle with making the right decisions when it comes to raising healthy and happy children as they attempt to find the best methods and techniques in a sea of misinformation. Parenting is mostly a balancing act, as you try to navigate your way through a sea of misinformation and bad advice. Some of the best advice is tried and true and has been so for generations. A lot of parenting styles and techniques over time have evolved to keep up with the ever-changing world. It can be incredibly difficult for a parent to decide on what's best for their kids.

This guide provides an extensive list of tips and critical pointers for parenting to be as smooth sailing as possible. Parents have testified to the efficacies of the advice in this book. More importantly, they are incredibly enthusiastic about how they have been able to get their own children on board to implement these habits into their lives willingly. Adhering to these tips and tricks, you will be on your way to successfully raising infants to teenagers and to fully thriving and capable adults. With recipes and activity ideas for you to try in your household, the techniques are simple to implement in your daily life but will benefit you and your children for years to come.

REFERENCES

Contento, I. (2008). Nutrition education: Linking research, theory, and practice. Asia Pac J Clin Nutr, 17(1), 176–179.

McGraw-Hill, & Parker, S.P. (2002). McGraw-Hill Dictionary of Scientific and Technical Terms, 6th edition, published by The McGraw-Hill Companies, Inc. Online: http://www.answers.com/library.

Rettner, R. (2012). Family Meals Help Kids Eat More Fruit & Veggies. Live Science, http://www.livescience.com/25700-family-meals-help-kidseat-more-fruit-veggies.html.

Bensley, R. J., Anderson, J. V., Brusk, J. J., Mercer, N., & Rivas, J. (2011). Impact of internet vs traditional Special Supplemental Nutrition

Program for Women, Infants, and Children nutrition education on fruit and vegetable intake. J Am Diet Assoc, 111(5), 749–755.

Neuenschwander, L. M., Abbott, A., & Mobleym, A. R. (2013). Comparison of a Web-Based vs In-Person Nutrition Education Program for LowIncome Adults. Journal of the Academy of Nutrition and Dietetics, 113(1), 120-126.

Random House Kernerman Webster's College Dictionary. (2010). K Dictionaries Ltd, by arrangement with Random House Information

Group,an imprint of The Crown Publishing Group, a division of Random House, Inc. Copyright 2005, 1997, 1991 by Random House, Online at: http://www.kdictionaries-online.com.

Bosma J. Development and impairments of feeding in infancy and childhood. In: Groher ME, ed. Dysphagia: Diagnosis and management. 3rd ed. Boston, MA: Butterworth-Heinemann; 1997:131-138.

Morris SE. Development of oral motor skills in the neurologically impaired child receiving non-oral feedings Dysphagia 1989;3:135-154.

Arimond M, Ruel MT. Dietary diversity is associated with child nutritional status: Evidence from 11 demographic and health surveys. The Journal of Nutrition 2004;134:2579-2585.

Skinner JD, Carruth BR, Bounds W, Ziegler P, Reidy K. Do food-related experiences in the first two years of life predict dietary variety in school-aged children? Journal of Nutrition Education and Behaviour 2002;34(6):310-315.

Schwartz C, Scholtens PA, Lalanne A, Weenen H, Nicklaus S. Development of healthy eating habits early in life. Review of recent evidence and selected guidelines. Appetite. 2011;57(3):796-807.

Mennella JA, Nicklaus S, Jagolino AL, Yourshaw LM. Variety is the spice of life: strategies for promoting fruit and vegetable acceptance during infancy. Physiol Behav. 2008;22;94(1):29-38.

Linscheid TR, Budd KS, Rasnake LK. Pediatric feeding disorders. In: Roberts MC, ed. Handbook of pediatric psychology. New York, NY: Guilford Press; 2003:481-498.

Birch LL, McPhee L, Shoba BC, Pirok E, Steinberg L. What kind of exposure reduces children's food neophobia? Looking vs tasting. Appetite 1987;9(3):171-178.

Keren M, Feldman R, Tyano S. Diagnoses and interactive patterns of infants referred to a community-based infant mental health clinic. Journal of the American Academy of Child & Adolescent Psychiatry 2001;40(1):27-35.

Palfreyman Z, Haycraft E, Meyer C. Development of the Parental Modeling of Eating Behaviours Scale (PARM): links with food intake among children and their mothers. Maternal and Child Nutrition. 2012 [Epub ahead of print].

Zoumas-Morse C, Rock CL, Sobo EJ, Neuhouser ML. Children's patterns of macronutrient intake and associations with restaurant and home eating. Journal of the American Dietetic Association 2001;101(8):923-925.

Smith MM, Lifshitz F. Excess fruit juice consumption as a contributing factor in nonorganic failure to thrive. Pediatrics 1994;93(3):438-443.

Ponza M, Devaney B, Ziegler P, Reidy K, Squatrito C. Nutrient intakes and food choices of infants and toddlers participating in WIC. Journal of the American Dietetic Association 2004;104(1 Suppl 1):71-79.

Devaney B, Kalb L, Briefel R, Zavitsky-Novak T, Clusen N, Ziegler P. Feeding infants and toddlers study: overview of the study design. Journal of the American Dietetic Association 2004;104(1 Suppl 1):8-13.

Picciano MF, Smiciklas-Wright H, Birch LL, Mitchell DC, Murray-Kolb L, McConahy KL. Nutritional guidance is needed during dietary transition in early childhood. Pediatrics 2000;106(1):109-114.

Cullen KW, Ash DM, Warneke C, de Moor C. Intake of soft drinks, fruit-flavored beverages, and fruits and vegetables by children in grades 4 through 6. American Journal of Public Health 2002;92(9):1475-1477.

Brotanek JM, Gosz J, Weitzman M, Flores G. Secular trends in the prevalence of iron deficiency among US toddlers, 1976-2002. Archives of Pediatrics & Adolescent Medicine 2008;162:374-81.

Ainsworth MDS, Blehar MC, Waters E, Wall S. Patterns of attachment: A psychological study of the strange situation. New York: Psychology Press, 1978.

Rhee K. Childhood overweight and the relationship between parent behaviors, parenting style, and family functioning. The Annals of the American Academy of Political and Social Science 2008;615:11–37.

Baumrind D. Rearing competent children In: Damon W, ed. Child development today and tomorrow. San Francisco, CA: Jossey-Bass Publishers; 1989:349-378.

Maccoby EE, Martin J. Socialization in the context of the family: parent-child interaction. In: Hetherington EM, ed. Handbook of child psychology: Socialization, personality, and social development. Vol 4. New York, NY: John Wiley; 1983:1-101.

Black MM & Aboud FE. Responsive feeding is embedded in a theoretical framework of responsive parenting. Journal of Nutrition 2011;141(3):490-4.

Like us on https://www.facebook.com/tcecpublishing/

http://www.thechildrenseducationcentre.co.uk/specialoffer

OTHER BOOKS YOU'LL LOVE!

CLICK ON THE BOOKS

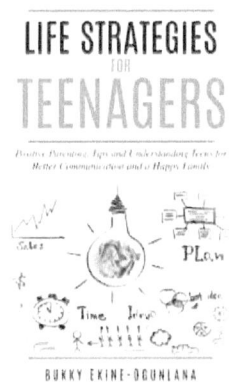

Link to Book

322 | OTHER BOOKS YOU'LL LOVE!

Link to Book

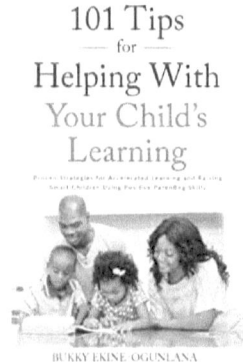

Link to Book

OTHER BOOKS YOU'LL LOVE! | 323

Link to Book

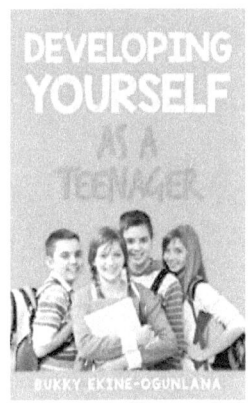

Link to Book

324 | OTHER BOOKS YOU'LL LOVE!

Link to Book

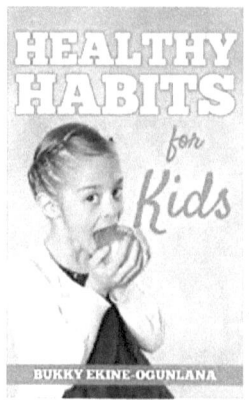

Link to Book

OTHER BOOKS YOU'LL LOVE! | 325

Link to Book

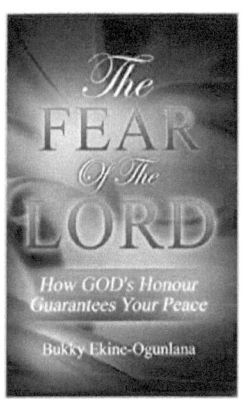

Link to Book

OTHER BOOKS YOU'LL LOVE!

Link to Book

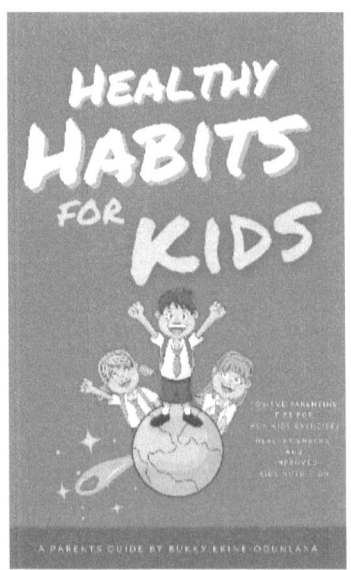

Link to Book

OTHER BOOKS YOU'LL LOVE! | 327

Link to Book

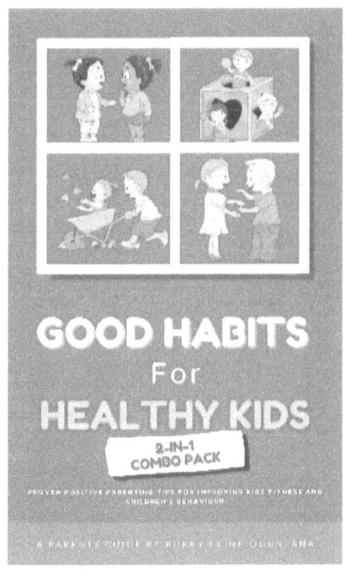

OTHER BOOKS YOU'LL LOVE!

[Link to Book](#)

www.ingramcontent.com/pod-product-compliance
Lightning Source LLC
Chambersburg PA
CBHW021139080526
44588CB00008B/125